AF866253

Norbert Elias and Sigmund Freud

This book explores the influence of Freudian psychoanalysis on Norbert Elias' theory of the civilizing process – an influence acknowledged by Elias himself – conducting a dialogue with a view to analyzing points of contact and distance between them. Examining the development of Elias' work, it sheds light on the integration of psychoanalytic concepts in his thought, considering the dynamics that exist between individuals and social processes, as the civilizing process affects the psychic economy of individuals and psychic structures serve to sustain civilization. A genealogical study of Freudian concepts as expressed in the trajectory of Elias's sociology, it will appeal to scholars of sociology and psychology with interests in social and psychoanalytic theory.

André Oliveira Costa is psychoanalyst, member of the Norbert Elias Foundation and the Psychoanalytic Association of Porto Alegre (APPOA), Brazil.

Classical and Contemporary Social Theory
Series Editor
Stjepan G. Mestrovic, *Texas A&M University, USA*

Classical and Contemporary Social Theory publishes rigorous scholarly work that re-discovers the relevance of social theory for contemporary times, demonstrating the enduring importance of theory for modern social issues. The series covers social theory in a broad sense, inviting contributions on both 'classical' and modern theory, thus encompassing sociology, without being confined to a single discipline. As such, work from across the social sciences is welcome, provided that volumes address the social context of particular issues, subjects, or figures and offer new understandings of social reality and the contribution of a theorist or school to our understanding of it.

The series considers significant new appraisals of established thinkers or schools, comparative works or contributions that discuss a particular social issue or phenomenon in relation to the work of specific theorists or theoretical approaches. Contributions are welcome that assess broad strands of thought within certain schools or across the work of a number of thinkers, but always with an eye toward contributing to contemporary understandings of social issues and contexts.

Titles in this series

Post-Philosophical Sociology
Eliasian Perspectives on the Sociology of Knowledge
Richard Kilminster

Exploring Emotions in Social Life
Michael Hviid Jacobsen

Vilfredo Pareto's Contributions to Modern Social Theory
Christopher Adair-Toteff

Norbert Elias and Sigmund Freud
The Psychoanalytic Foundations of the Civilizing Process
André Oliveira Costa

For more information about this series, please visit: www.routledge.com/sociology/series/ASHSER1383

Norbert Elias and Sigmund Freud

The Psychoanalytic Foundations of the Civilizing Process

André Oliveira Costa

Routledge
Taylor & Francis Group
LONDON AND NEW YORK

First published 2024
by Routledge
4 Park Square, Milton Park, Abingdon, Oxon OX14 4RN

and by Routledge
605 Third Avenue, New York, NY 10158

Routledge is an imprint of the Taylor & Francis Group, an informa business

© 2024 André Oliveira Costa

The right of André Oliveira Costa to be identified as author of this work has been asserted in accordance with sections 77 and 78 of the Copyright, Designs and Patents Act 1988.

All rights reserved. No part of this book may be reprinted or reproduced or utilised in any form or by any electronic, mechanical, or other means, now known or hereafter invented, including photocopying and recording, or in any information storage or retrieval system, without permission in writing translated by Lisa Shaw the publishers.

Trademark notice: Product or corporate names may be trademarks or registered trademarks, and are used only for identification and explanation without intent to infringe.

British Library Cataloguing-in-Publication Data
A catalogue record for this book is available from the British Library

ISBN: 978-1-032-45843-4 (hbk)
ISBN: 978-1-032-45846-5 (pbk)
ISBN: 978-1-003-37893-8 (ebk)

DOI: 10.4324/9781003378938

Typeset in Times New Roman
by Apex CoVantage, LLC

To Alice and Maíra.

Contents

1 The court and the civilization

Norbert Elias was born on 22 June 1987, in Breslau, a small town that then belonged to Prussia, and today is located in Poland and named Wrocław. Elias died in Amsterdam in 1990 at the age of 93, on the 1 August 1990. The only son of a Jewish merchant couple, he spent his childhood and adolescence in that town, until the outbreak of World War I, when he applied to join the army and was sent to the front. His mother, Sophie, frequented Jewish society circles while his father, Hermann, was a successful businessman in the textile industry, a Prussian that, as Elias recalled, had a moustache that imitated that of the emperor. His father, sitting on the sofa, reflecting with his index finger against his nose, immersed in his own thoughts, never escaped his memory and the very way Elias himself used to put himself when he put himself to thinking. Elias participated in World War I as a soldier in a communications unit, being responsible for the installation of telephone lines. After the end of the war, he returned to his native town and enrolled on undergraduate courses in both medicine and philosophy, soon abandoning the latter. In 1925, after having submitted a doctoral thesis in philosophy, titled *Idea and individual: a critical investigation of the notion of history* [*Idee und Individuum. Eine kritische Untersuchung zum Begriff der Geschichte*], at the University of Breslau, he moved to Heidelberg to work as an assistant to Karl Mannheim.

His move to the University of Heidelberg and his work with Mannheim at the Institute of Social and Political Sciences [*Institut für Sozial und Staatswissenschaften*], between 1924 and 1930, was a formative period, giving him the cultural background required for the development of an ambitious and original project. The change of city also contributed to his break with philosophical and metaphysical thought and, in particular, with the neo-Kantian influences of his thesis supervisor, Richard Hönigswald. In that period, Elias was close to a group of politicized students, who gathered around Marianne and Alfred Weber, wife and brother of the sociologist Max Weber, knowing that it would be impossible to conduct any intellectual work if he continued to adopt the perspective of the isolated individual, as was the norm in traditional philosophy.

In the early 1930s, Elias moved to the University of Frankfurt, accompanying his professor, who was appointed to the chair of sociology. According to Elias (2014), in an interview with Johan Heilbron, in Frankfurt psychoanalysis was part of the *décor* and had a close relationship with sociology. Together with Marxist

DOI: 10.4324/9781003378938-1

theory, which was already consolidated within university culture, Freudian thought constituted one of the central tenets of social science research. Consequently, Elias positioned himself intellectually between university Marxism and an attempt to adapt Freudian thought to a psycho-social context, where he could propose a sociology that could try to solve the problem of the imbrication of social processes and personality structures.

In Frankfurt, Elias witnessed the creation of two great institutions, for which psychoanalysis was an important reference: the Institute for Social Research [*Institut für Sozialforschung*], created by Max Horkheimer and Theodor Adorno, which gave rise to the well-known the *Frankfurt School*, and the Psychoanalytic Institute of Frankfurt [*Frankfurter Psychoanalytisches Institut*], created by Karl Landauer and Heinrich Meng in 1929, which would play host to psychoanalysts like Otto Fenichel, S.H. Foulkes, the couple Erich Fromm and Frieda Fromm-Reichmann, Clara Happel and Herbert Marcuse. In that same interview Elias reported that his relationship with Adorno and Horkheimer was extremely courteous, but also one of mutual scorn. Not exactly directed towards him, but especially to his professor Mannheim, who considered them doctrinaire Marxists, while being seen by them as a semi-bourgeois leftist. In any case, all of them occupied the same physical space, sharing the same rooms in the Institute for Social Research, and forming an environment that stimulated intellectual reflection, theoretical debate and a critical position that revised the canonical thoughts of the time.

In 1933 Elias turned to researching the configuration of court society, aiming to understand how the constitution of the modern state (in this case, the absolutist French state of the XVI to XVIII centuries) was linked to the psychic economies of the individual. Despite the results of that research being published for the first time in 1969, under the title *The Court Society* [*Die höfische Gesellschaft*], it was one of his first works, establishing dialogues with his main references, the economic-philosophical work of Karl Marx and the sociology of Max Weber. His research about the society of the French court of the *Ancien Régime* was to serve as a habilitation thesis for the position of *Privatdozent* at the University of Frankfurt. The writing of that project, entitled initially *The man of the court* [*Der höfische Mensch*] could not be presented because at that time the German National Socialist Party had just taken power, and Elias was forced to exile.

1.1 The desire for distinction and the fetish of prestige

The importance of Sigmund Freud's psychoanalysis in the work of Norbert Elias was acknowledged several times by the sociologist himself, according to his statement to the *Libération* newspaper, on 5 December 1985: "Without Freud, I would not be able to write what I wrote. His theory was essential for my work and all his concepts (ego, superego, libido etc.) are very familiar to me" (Elias 1985: 92). Throughout his work, Elias's return to psychoanalysis to elaborate some foundations of his theory on civilizing process, thinking that civilization is moving towards the internalization of mechanisms of self-control through the repression of drives. Even though the influence of psychoanalysis had a forceful, but also silent, influence on the sociologist, this did not prevent him from positioning himself as a severe critic of Sigmund Freud's thought. Thus, in a follow-up to that interview, he establishes some of his objections to Freudian theory:

> But Freud, throughout all his life, studied men and women that lived in the late XIX century and early XX century, and – in the vogue of the natural sciences – he forged his concepts as if the structure of the personality that he was observing was that of all human beings.
>
> (Elias 1985: 92)

Elias's disagreement with Freud's research stems from the psychoanalyst attributing a "universal value to a given and dated type of personality structure" (Elias 1985: 92). Freud formulated, according to the sociologist, a concept of the individual who did not consider the transformations and changes experienced by different social formations throughout the centuries. Because of that, according to his critique, psychoanalysis could not understand the transformations of man throughout history, explaining psychopathologies in terms of immutable and atemporal structures.

In a continuation of this interview, Elias explains that, starting by identifying certain limitations of psychoanalysis, it was necessary "to go beyond Freud", that is,

> to recognize the transformations that affected the development of human personality and to think that in a world where knowledge about the natural world was not ours, where fears and anxieties were obsessive, the structure of personality could not be that of the men of the XX century. So, the need to employ terms and concepts other than Freud's to characterize former psychic economies. For instance, we cannot talk about a superego of medieval man. The problem is to understand how and why the structure of personality that is described by Freud emerged progressively.
>
> (Elias 1985: 92)

Norbert Elias' sociology builds on and goes beyond the concepts and ideas of psychoanalysis, turning to the psychic transformations that took place within social processes. This means that Elias's work recognizes that psychoanalysis is a theory of the mind that should be rooted in a consideration of the processes of transformation within social structures and because of this, seeks to go beyond Freud's ideas. In his book *The Civilizing Process. Sociogenetic and Psychogenetic Investigations* [*Über den Prozeß der Zivilisation. Soziogenetische und psychogenetische Untersuchungen*], Elias states: "It may be 'that there have always been' 'neuroses'. But the 'neuroses' we see about us today are a specific historical form of psychic conflict which needs psychogenetic and sociogenetic illumination" (Elias 1939: 127). It is in this sense that it is possible to grasp one of Elias's propositions to trace the sociogenesis of psychic structures, that is, to investigate the social conditions that led to the psychic processes of the unconscious. This project took Elias beyond the scope of psychoanalytical research, but also beyond the very current sociological thought of the time, involving sociogenesis and psychogenesis.

In October 1987, Elias gave an interview for the German television network ZDF, published later in the book *I followed my own path: a route through the century* [*J'ai suivi mon propre chemin: un parcours dans le siècle*]. When asked about his sources of inspiration, about who influenced his thinking in decisive ways, he again made reference to Freudian psychoanalysis:

> Among the individual works that influenced me, I could only truly mention the work of Freud. Freud's psychoanalytic theory had, as a theory, a strong influence over my work. I cannot mention any other work, or specific book that has had a comparable influence on me.
>
> (Elias 1987: 69)

Even if Freud was the most important theoretician for his thinking, Elias does not forget to mention, in that interview, the importance of Karl Marx, as well as his advisor, Karl Mannheim, and that of Theodor Adorno and Max Horkheimer, founders of the *Frankfurt School*. What Freud and Adorno did, according to Elias, was elevate the repression of individuals to the level of human universality. However, contrary to the proposal to think about the psychic economy in terms of long-term social transformations, these authors, in Elias's opinion, seemed to consider what was happening in Vienna and Frankfurt as a paradigm of humanity.

The initial period of his intellectual formation allowed the German sociologist the freedom to work in an innovative and creative way (Joly 2012), making progress with a sociological proposal that included both social dynamics and unconscious psychic processes. He suggested thinking about Freud's psychoanalysis in the light of social processes, while he turned a critical eye to the theoretical sociological tradition, adding subjective processes to its precepts in the search for a way of thinking that could value the individual psychic mechanisms in connection with social processes. Elias's relationship with psychoanalysis did not restrict itself to theoretical issues because being one of the founders of the Group Analytic Society, he actively collaborated in the development of group psychotherapy together with the German psychoanalyst Siegmund H. Foulkes. Moreover, on a personal level, he carried out his didactic analysis with Kate Friedlander, a Jewish psychoanalyst who left Germany in 1933 and became a disciple of Anna Freud in England.

In the same way that Norbert Elias questioned the connection between the individual and society, Sigmund Freud also sought to go beyond this relation as if it were an antinomy to the point of identifying the superego as a psychic entity that marks the internalization of social rules. Along with the idea that civilization is established on the repression of drives, the appropriation of that concept by Elias was fundamental for the development of his theory of the civilizing process. Finally, in Freud (1930), the theory of cultural discontents determined the conditions for the possibility of social ties for Norbert Elias. This hypothesis also had an impact on Elias, in that even if making reference to terms such as *process* and *civilization* during World War II and in the context of attempts to exterminate the

Jewish people, he never failed to point out the discontents produced by the encounter between individuals.

The book *The Court Society* sets out to investigate French court society of the *Ancien Régime* as a specific type of social configuration seen from the perspective of social and psychological processes, which means that changes in social relations occur in continuity with transformations in the psychic economy of individuals. In that work, Elias considers that the court and the members of the court form an inseparable whole: "Court society is not a phenomenon that exists outside the individuals forming it; the individuals forming it, whether the king or the valet, do not exist outside the society which they form together" (Elias 1969: 18). In the introduction that he wrote for the first edition of the book, in 1969, points out that at the time he was developing this research, he already proposed to think about the imbrication of individual processes with social structures, a project he carried out throughout his entire life, going beyond the concepts that characterize the terms individual and society as autonomous and independent.

Elias stressed his intention to position himself against the dichotomic positions that sustained the society as extra-individual and the individual as extra-social. This meant that Elias's criticisms were directed at the claims to scientificity of areas like psychology, sociology, and history that treat their objects as if they were independent. "Individual" and "society" are, then, two concepts that should not be taken as mutually exclusive and independent objects, but as processes that differ from each other and are at the same time indissociable. To understand court society as a social formation in constant motion, Elias sought to analyze the dynamics of this structure by investigating the relationship between sociogenetic and psychogenetic processes, showing how the formation of court society constituted particular social and psychological dynamics. In Elias's words,

> The concepts "individual" and "society" are often used as if they referred to two different substances at rest. These terms can easily give the impression that they denote not only different objects, but objects existing in absolute isolation from one another. But in reality it is to processes that these words refer, processes that can be distinguished but not separated. The king's personal development and that of his position go hand in hand.
>
> (Elias 1969: 20)

In *The Court Society*, Elias presents some fundamental concepts underpinning his work, such as configuration, interdependence, and equilibrium of tensions so that through them, it is possible to understand that "How and why people are bound together to form specific dynamic configurations is one of the central questions, perhaps even the central question, of sociology" (Elias 1969: 208). The concept of *configuration*, based on which Elias's work is often referred to as *configurational sociology*, qualifies a relation of *interdependence* and *power* between the members of a society and explains how changes in a given social formation are concomitant with changes in the psychic economy of individuals. He begins with the principle that people are born in a multiplicity of mutual dependences, forming part of a network of invisible bonds that condition the actions and the affections of each person. Society, in turn, also is dependent on the actions of individuals, forming networks of different types of relations.

Thus, through the formulation of such a concept as configuration, Elias can overcome not only the antithesis between the individual and society, but also the separation of different historical periods, showing that a society that configures itself as certain modes of social relations maintains itself even after certain changes over generations, transmitting experiences in the form of *socially acquired knowledge*, whose origins lose their meaning and become unknown to those who reproduce them. That is, individuals internalize and reproduce ways of being, thinking and behaving that are specific to certain figurations that are transmitted to their descendants without the latter being aware of their motives or intentions.

The legacy from one social figuration to another indicates that something of these ancient societies remain preserved, as one can deduce from the following explanation given by Elias:

> As a central figuration of that stage of development, which after a long struggle gave way abruptly or gradually to a professional-bourgeois-urban-industrial stage, this aristocratic court society developed a civilizing and cultural physiognomy which was taken over by professional- bourgeois society partly as a heritage and partly as an antithesis and, preserved in this way, was further developed. By studying the structure of court society and seeking to understand one of the last great non-bourgeois figurations of the West, therefore, we indirectly gain increased understanding of our own professional-bourgeois, urban-industrial society.
>
> (Elias 1969: 40)

It is in the perspective of understanding which elements of the courtly *ethos* were preserved in later societies that we turn to this study. One can find in this period not only a genesis of our contemporary society, but also a genesis of the psychic economy as we know it presented by the psychoanalytic investigations of Sigmund Freud. In this sense, the dynamics of the configuration of court societies will help us to understand the dynamics of unconscious psychic structures and processes.

Thus, one can understand that the court society did not disappear over time but was preserved and was transmitted to other social configurations, reproducing itself in the establishment of *social habitus* in each individual. Or rather, different social configurations repeat hegemonic patterns of behaviour from ancient societies. The difference between the customs of the court aristocracy and those of the bourgeoisie established particular social *ethos* for each of these social strata. Bourgeois, obliged to guarantee the success of their lives through success at work and having to hand over their income to the family's expenses, lived always thinking about the need to save to guarantee the future. The way of acting of industrial-bourgeois societies was organized by the control of behaviours and emotions according to the professional life of each individual, forming a bourgeois *ethos* markedly controlled by the economy. The court aristocrats, on the other hand, in their search for ostentation and wealth, had their *ethos* marked by the "consumption of prestige", by recognition and status determined by the eyes of others.

The concept of configuration is the starting point for an analytical methodology for examining social processes that never treats its object as an isolated or autonomous entity, but always as interdependent regarding other social processes. In the case of court society, it supports a sociological theory of interdependence in which each individual seeks to attain values of prestige, status, and importance from the higher classes, engendering constant battles and competitions, in a balance of tensions that can never be resolved. A relation of power underlies the relation between the individual, who fights to belong to higher social levels, at the same time as feeling threatened by those that belong to the lower levels of society. Elias says,

> The desire to stand out, to distinguish oneself socially from those who do not belong, finds its linguistic expression in terms like *valeur*, *considération*, *se distinguer*, and in many others which, used as a matter of course, are both a shibboleth of membership and proof of respect for the same social ideals.
> (Elias 1969: 65 – emphasis in original)

In this logic of the distinction of the court society, distinction, and competition barriers between the social classes were established in court society so that necessarily one group will lose and be excluded from access to better social opportunities. An analysis of the social transformations of that period that extends from the Middle Ages up to the formation of the modern state, reveals a rationale that was directed towards the regulation of the affects and feelings that each individual exerts on himself and on others. The court acted on individuals, for example, in accordance with a rational logic organized around assessments of the layout of places of social circulation in dwellings (*hôtels*, *palais*, *châteaux*, etc.); around ceremonies that involved courtiers, like the *lever* and the *coucher* of the king and the queen; and around the etiquette rules that regulated glances, body movements, affections, and the way to deal with other people and that established positions of power and excluded any other ways of thinking, feeling, and behaving that did not fit within their conceptions.

The court was not only a society for individuals. It was the very condition of their existence. It was not a representation or an act, but the actual reality. Furthermore, it was from it that they understood the world, that they established the circle of distance and proximities between the different social classes, that they determined who was superior or belonged to the lower classes. Their lives depended on the social recognition and privileges that other people gave them.

> In court society, it was meaningful for a duke to be a duke, for a count to be a count, and for every bearer of court privilege to bear such privilege. Every threat to the privileged position of a single house, as to the system of privileges in general, was a threat to what gave value and meaning to the people of this society in their own eyes and in those of others around them whose opinions mattered for them. Every loss of privilege meant a loss of meaning and purpose.
> (Elias 1969: 76)

Insofar as public relationships determined the meaning of life for each person, it was necessary to establish rigorous distinctions between the different social classes. The individuals who had to work to sustain themselves were situated outside the *grand monde*, at the margins of society. Individuals who belonged to the high circles of the court received more prestige and recognition from others. Thus, life in the court had to be based on lust, riches, pleasure, and amusements. Paradoxically, however, the fiercest restrictions were imposed on the courtesans, for their lives depended on physical appearances, the state of their houses, the refinement of their posture, language, and behaviour.

As Elias describes, court society was organized in unstable balances of power in which each member, including the king, established relations of dependence with others. The king, therefore, was also dependent on power games, assigning or withdrawing privileges to control the nobles closest to him to maintain the nobility as a distinct class separate from the others. Insofar as the king was the only individual at court who did not suffer forces from all sides, but only those from below, he used etiquette as an instrument of domination to maintain the balance of tensions and thereby secure his own place of privilege. The king, as well as or more than the other courtiers, was not free from the forces the ceremonial etiquette and external coercions that he himself imposed on his subjects: "He could not subject other people to ceremony and display as mean of power without subjecting himself to them as well" (Elias 1969: 136), says Elias.

In the formation of court societies, a regulating principle limits and directs spontaneous behaviours and affections, establishing a more complex society, more differentiated and with a greater degree of dependence among its members. Each person increasingly controls and is controlled, watches and is watched, scolds and is scolded. Power is not a property that the individual possesses, but an attribute of value in human relations that does not allow them to be homogeneous or harmonious. Therefore, the tensions and conflicts produced by power games lead to the establishment of distinctions and, consequently, of social exclusions between established groups and marginal groups, as was the case between the nobles and the bourgeoisie within court society.

An analysis of the transition between the feudal period and the formation of the French absolutist state shows that the civilizing process led to greater individuation and differentiation of individuals, as well as to them establishing between themselves more enduring, more complex, and more stable networks of interdependence. In court societies, the life of each person depended on his attitudes and on what others may think of them. The identity of each individual was constituted through the eyes of others. Without that social opinion, his life made no sense. Social opinion was "the foundation of existence" (Elias 1969: 95), says Elias. An *ethos* of court society began to be formed, marked by what Elias calls the *fetish-prestige*, regulating etiquettes and ceremonials, distribution, and circulation in the public and private spaces of housing, and the balance of tensions among its members. Everyone was bound by court rationality, acting out of obligation to the extent that external coercions had not yet been internalized in individuals. Any behaviour or expression of emotion that did not comply with the norms and rules of the ceremonials were subject to threats of demotion in social hierarchy, of loss of power and favours, and even removal from the social circle.

> In the last analysis this compelling struggle for ever-threatened power and prestige was the dominant factor that condemned all those involved to enact these burdensome ceremonies. No single person within the figuration was able to initiate a reform of the tradition.
>
> (Elias 1969: 87)

Any change in the unstable balance of power between the different classes of the aristocracy threatened all those who belonged to the complex chain of interdependence. Thus, no one appreciated any kind of change, running the risk of feeling outside the social circle, or even feeling excluded by the creation of a new rule. Labels and moral rules produced hierarchical spaces of belonging and non-belonging to social groups. Members of the court identified with the *ethos* of the nobility kept themselves distanced from other hierarchically inferior individuals, who occupied places within other courts or were outside them, to stay within the circles of privilege and social recognition, according to Elias:

> The courtier had no possibility of changing place, leaving Paris or Versailles and continuing his life elsewhere without loss of prestige or self-respect. Only in this one court society could its members preserve what gave them direction and purpose in their own eyes, their social existence as court people, their aloofness from all else, their prestige – the centre of their self-image and of their personal identity.
>
> (Elias 1969: 99)

Differences in etiquette, habits, and behaviour produced hierarchical relations among the courtiers themselves, establishing different positions of power and prestige, as well as who could be part of this or that social circle. Everyone's existence depended on the opinion that others had about them. Identification with social class marked the identity of the individual so that the loss of that social position could even mean death. Everything revolved around the court, the social position the individual occupied, and the value he achieved among others. Each individual was subject to the eyes of everyone. Elias continues,

> They went to court not only because they were dependent on the king; they remained dependent on the king because it was only by going to court and living within court society that they could preserve the distance from everything else on which their spiritual salvation, their prestige as court aristocrats, in short, their social existence and their personal identity depended.
>
> (Elias 1969: 99)

The *fetish-prestige*, which often resulted in conflicts between the inferior and the superior social classes, established court habits that instrumentalized the art of dealing with people through the elaboration of ever more complex rules of coercion for behaviour and affections. The rigorous obedience of norms, the precision of the gestures at each ceremony, the adequate expression of emotions, all such factors were not formalities of social interaction, but rather necessary and vital for those that frequented the court. Court society forged a social mechanism powered by competition, in which people depended on all kinds of coercions and regulatory calculations. Controls on other also meant controlling yourself. In the words of Elias, "This self-observation and the observation of the other people are complementary" (Elias 1969: 105). To differentiate themselves from others, people regulated themselves, shaped by the gaze of others, who observed every aspect of behaviour and every feeling.

Habits placed the individual in a given position within a specific social hierarchy, and at the same time established differences between each other and all those who were strangers to the group. More than an empty formality, etiquette was an instrument of control and power. It was through etiquette, says Elias, that hierarchization between social classes expressed itself in the most conspicuous way. Social coercion served precisely to establish social differences between aristocrats and provincial nobles, as well as the administrative nobility and the people. The way each person behaved represented the prestige that she received in the opinion of the others. For that reason, in each ceremony and in each expression of affection, there was a minimal margin for any type of spontaneous and unexpected manifestation.

All this was sustained via a rationale specific to court society, where what stood out was the concern with himself, with his own interests, the privileges and recognitions that guaranteed a certain place within a social hierarchy and even made possible his existence within this space. All these dynamics, we can say, forged a kind of sociogenesis of the narcissism, when courtiers had to start to dam a certain amount of psychic energy within themselves in order not to decompensate the balance of the interdependent social relations of which they were part of: "It was not only in the sphere of bourgeois capitalist competition that the idea of egoism as a motive of human action was formed, but first of all in the completion of the court " (Elias 1969: 105). In the art of *observing* people, in the art of *describing* people, in the art of *dealing* with people, in the art of *controlling* gestures and emotions, through all of these behaviour there was a process of self-observation, an immersion in one's own interiority that did not represent an immersion into the depths of personality, but a form of control over oneself in order to protect oneself from any threat caused by any rupture with the standards of etiquette.

> Why this attitude becomes important to court people is easily seen: affective outbursts are difficult to control and calculate. They reveal the true feelings of the person concerned to a degree that, because not calculated, can be damaging; they hand over trump cards to rivals for favour and prestige. Above all, they are a sign of weakness.
>
> (Elias 1969: 111)

The rationale of the court – of the precise calculation, of control and rigidity, of predictability and precaution, of good taste and elegance, of social convention and competition for prestige – remains mixed with forms of bourgeois and capitalist rationality. What was created in one configuration does not disappear when it is transformed into a new configuration, but remains preserved in the forgetting of its origins. For Elias, the court *ethos* did not disappear with the extinction of this figuration or with the emergence of other figurations, but was passed on to them under other guises:

> But elements of the estate ethos that we distinguish – by the example of court motivation through "honour" or "prestige" – from the economic ethos of bourgeois strata, can permeate the latter ethos under certain conditions. As soon as exclusive, elitist tendencies appear in bourgeois strata, they also express themselves in prestige symbols directed at maintaining the group's distance from others, while transfiguring its existence.
>
> (Elias 1969: 103)

The problem that runs through *The Court Society* is describing a particular form of power distribution, whose structures were renewed over the generations, transmitting to new individuals the habits of a society marked by the forgetting of its origins. Elias continues,

> Nevertheless, many of the forms that the court society of those centuries imparted to people and their environment, whether it be furniture, pictures or clothes, forms of greeting or social etiquette, theatre, poetry or houses, live on in the nineteenth and twentieth centuries. But it was a peculiarly ghostly transformation that the heritage of court society underwent in the bourgeois age. This heritage was coarsened in a specific way by the new mass society and emptied of its original meaning.
>
> (Elias 1969: 113–114)

Part of the court rationale was transmitted and inherited by the new configuration of industrial and bourgeois societies, founding the rationality of economic values with marks of the good society. In the same way, it transferred to the background of the private life of individuals and, little by little, to the background of the psychic life, the conflicts and antagonisms that occupied the centre of the tensions of court society.

The ability to submit to etiquette indicates the human value of each individual, whether he was an inferior or superior being to others, whether he belonged to good society or whether he was on the margins of the *grand monde*. More than a way of life that sought to be recognized by luxury and ostentation, the *fetish-prestige* manifested the meaning of each person's existence. As a consequence, the quest to remain within the circle of the favoured ones of the court produced power struggles and competition games between social classes. The fear of losing one's place in the sun, of no longer being part of the privileged life at court, and of no longer being recognized by the king or one's equals led each individual to engage in empty ceremonial, to submit to rules of etiquette, and to internalize inconsistent habits.

1.2 The paradoxes of the court and social anxiety

In the context of the formation of court society, individuals were being compelled to renounce the satisfaction of their drives, internalizing habits and manners to live peacefully in more complex and stable societies. During this process, external social coercions were gradually transferred to the backstage of psychic life. The use of a civilizing mask, a mask of coercions that individuals used to related to each other, demanded self-regulation in the way they thought, felt, and behaved. Consequently, a new social grammar was reorganizing the drive economy of individuals in a new form of discontent in civilization. Elias says,

> In court society the armour is not yet all-embracing and automatic as in these working societies, since the greater inequality of people, the subjection, dependence and submissiveness of the lower-ranking, particularly the poorer strata, always open a broad social field to court people in which affective impulses of all kinds can be relatively openly expressed without being threatened by social failure or penalties, and within which, therefore, the development of self-constraint is only slightly demanded. For this reason the armour of the court aristocracy is by and large fairly loose. Court aristocrats are often well aware that they wear a mask in their dealings with other people, even though they may not be aware that playing with masks has become second nature to them.
>
> (Elias 1969: 241)

The need to escape from the oppressions of the civilizing process projected places of utopias, where individuals could rediscover the truth that had been undermined from themselves. It is a problem that the man of the court society, eager to escape the strong coercion imposed by civilization, cannot solve without destroying the social distinctions that put him in a superior position to others and that give value and meaning to his life without, at the same time, destroying himself. With a certain melancholization of the social bond, court society turned its eyes to finding a life free of coercion, where it could live simply and peacefully, and where it would be easier to satisfy the desires and achieve the pleasures that were no longer possible in a courtly life. Through the relationship with nature, life in the countryside came to represent a lost, more innocent and truer life, untethered from civilizing obligations. The idealization of peasant life, supposed to be more independent and more spontaneous in affections and behaviours, pointed to a way of being of individuals that was no longer found within the society of the court and the urban centres that were being formed. Elias continues,

> In the age of transition, nobles who had grown up on the estates of their ancestors had to accustom themselves to the more refined and diverse court life, with its more complex relationships that demanded far greater self-control. Even in these generations, the country life and scenery of their youth became

> for many men and women of the court an object of melancholy longing... Country life became a symbol of lost innocence, of spontaneous simplicity and naturalness. It became an opposite image to urban court life with its greater constraints, its more complex hierarchical pressures and its heavier demands on individual self-control.
>
> (Elias 1969: 223)

Life in past times, represented in periods of antiquity, also began to be a time of utopia, of realizing ideals of happiness, as a moment when one could rediscover an existence left behind. According to Elias,

> One of the forms in which they [feelings] can find symbolic expression is the projection of one's own ideals into the dream-image of a better, freer, more natural life in the past. The peculiarly romantic light in which this bathes the past, the light of an unrealizable longing, an unattainable ideal, a love that cannot be fulfilled, is the reflection of the conflict discussed earlier, the conflict of people who cannot destroy the constraints from which they suffer – whether they arise from the power structure or from civilization or a combination of the two – without destroying the foundation and the distinguishing mark of their high social position, what gives their lives meaning and value in their own eyes – without destroying themselves.
>
> (Elias 1969: 229)

Childhood life also begins to be represented as a utopian place, with nostalgia for a freer, more natural age, without the weight of coercion. "[The courtier] could return to the home of his ancestors but would not be able to find there what he sought. The free country existence of his childhood has become a dream like his childhood itself" (Elias 1969: 229), says Elias.

Many years later, at the age of 86 and almost blind, Norbert Elias described the effects of the transition of European society between an aristocratic society, which practiced leisure at court, and a bourgeois society, dedicated to work and money, in a short essay entitled *Watteau's Pilgrimage to the Isle of Love*. Elias takes as his object of analysis the painting "Pilgrimage to the Island of Citera", painted by Antoine Watteau in 1712, where we see the scene of couples in love leaving, in a utopian flight from political ideals, to the island of Citera, the island of love. Watteau's painting became the representation of a lost paradise, of a time when life was all about love trips and elegant balls, like an eternal dream of a life of pleasures. However, says Elias, the conflict between ideal and reality produces disillusionment. And, in this way, the transition from a utopia of ideals gave way to a utopia of pessimism, of lamenting the lost dream. The predominance of utopias of ideals, then, was slowly replaced by the predominance of utopias of fear and anxiety.

Thus, from the 15th century until the 19th century, individuals repeatedly found in this utopia an appropriate instrument to give vent to their desires, to their yearning for greater freedom from the coercions that imprison love. But until the end of the 18th century, as it transpired, it was mainly from social pressures that one sought to escape through the ideal image of the pilgrimage to the island of the pagan goddess. In the 19th century, another kind of pressures entered the scene, stronger than ever in the field of literary and artistic attention: people's internal pressures.

In this context, Norbert Elias, in *The Court Society*, cites three fundamental actions within the civilizing process that we cannot but associate with the three sources of human suffering identified by Freud, in *Civilization and Its Discontents* [*Das Unbehagen in der Kultur*]. According to the sociologist, there was the control exercised over "extra-human Nature, the control of people over each other, and the control of each individual over himself" (Elias 1969: 221). In turn, Freud, in this text published only three years before Elias, returned to the research of the court societies, points out that the discontents of our civilization stems from contact with three sources that erupt against the individual:

> We are threatened with suffering from three directions: from our own body, which is doomed to decay and dissolution and which cannot even do without pain and anxiety as warning signals; from the external world, which may rage against us with overwhelming and merciless forces of destruction; and finally from our relations to other men.
>
> (Freud 1930: 77)

As an effect of the civilizing process, Freud described discontent in civilization as the impossibility for individuals to control the forces of *nature*, to bear the relationship with *others*, whose suffering is the most painful of all, and to admit the fragility of their own *body*, which is commanded by uncontrollable desires and drives. From his investigations of court society, then, Norbert Elias presents us with a sociogenesis of discontent in civilization In 1930, Freud already pointed out the correspondence between the development of libido in the individual and in social processes, so that in both drive remnants that were not symbolized remain preserved and are unconsciously transmitted throughout the generations: "what is past in mental life *may* be preserved and is not *necessarily* destroyed" (Freud 1930: 71). The experiences that were inscribed in the unconscious long ago are not destroyed, but preserved as a memory that has been forgotten. The older structures are absorbed into the later phases without, however, being erased or abandoned. It was Norbert Elias who said that these remnants of the drive are transformed by the civilizing process into habits and customs, which end up having their origins forgotten and their intentions denied.

In the centre of Freudian theory of discontent in civilization, helplessness is its primary condition. The ego's condition of the psychic helplessness makes it completely dependent on others for its survival. The child, feeling protected and realizing that someone else is meeting his needs, begins to be able to establish affective bonds with his caregiver. In this sense, not only the need to survive, but also the need for protection and love makes individuals establish a relationship of dependency with others. Love and protection are initially imbricated. The loss of one could imply the loss of the other. As Freud states in *Civilization and Its Discontents*,

> If he loses the love of a person upon whom he is dependent, he also ceases to be protected from a variety of dangers. Above all, he is exposed to the danger that this stronger person will show his superiority in the form of punishment.
> (Freud 1930: 124)

It is therefore necessary to avoid the loss of love in order to maintain protection. The feeling of guilt, which before could be produced by the fear of being discovered for a wrong done, then became an unconscious mechanism of control by the individual's own relationship with internalized authority. Thus, as indicated by Freud, the distinction between *doing* and *desiring* is lost, to the extent that not even thinking can escape the criticism of the superego.

> Originally, renunciation of instinct was the result of fear of an external authority: one renounced one's satisfactions in order not to lose its love. If one has carried out this renunciation, one is, as it were, quits with the authority and no sense of guilt should remain. But with fear of the super ego the case is different. Here, instinctual renunciation is not enough, for the wish persists and cannot be concealed from the super ego. Thus, in spite of the renunciation that has been made, a sense of guilt comes about. This constitutes a great economic disadvantage in the erection of a super-ego, or, as we may put it, in the formation of a conscience. Instinctual renunciation now no longer has a completely liberating effect; virtuous continence is no longer rewarded with the assurance of love. A threatened externa unhappiness – loss of love and punishment on the part of the external authority – has been exchanged for a permanent internal unhappiness, for the tension of the sense of guilt.
> (Freud 1930: 127–128)

First, one renounces the drives for fear of being attacked or losing the love of external authority: "love is a protection against this punitive aggression" (Freud 1930: 128). Then authority is established in the form of moral consciousness – the superego – and renunciation to drives follows the fear that turns to it. Fear, at that moment, becomes that of the loss of love of the internal authority, but on the condition that it is no longer possible to differentiate a bad *intention* from a bad *action*. Thinking and acting receive the same value of reality for the unconscious and, most of the time, psychic reality gains the status effective reality. It is in the need to be in accordance with the rules imposed by the superego where the origin of discontent in civilization is to be found. The fear of the loss of love and protection translates into *anxiety* or *social fear*, insofar as the individual can no longer escape from internalized social coercion.

At the 25th conference of the *Introductory Conferences to Psychoanalysis* [*Die Einführung in die Psychoanalyse*], held between 1916 and 1917, Freud resumes the idea that the primordial condition of the ego is one of psychic and biological helplessness, making the newborn baby completely dependent on the help of the other to survive. In his early days, the ego feels threatened as much by external dangers as by internal dangers, coming from uncontrollable driving forces. Gradually, he establishes defence mechanisms against both, so that, relating to the first, withdrawal becomes a possible escape, while faced with the second, repression protects him through the formation of symptoms.

What Freud calls reality anxiety [*Realangst*] represents the condition of helplessness in the face of a situation that endangers the self-preservation of individuals. In the case of an *infant*, the danger arises in the absence of the other who can protect him and satisfy his vital needs:

> We may say of it that it is a reaction to the perception of external danger – that is, of an injury which is expected and foreseen. It is connected with the flight reflex and may be regarded as a manifestation of the self-preservative instinct.
>
> (Freud 1916–1917c: 394)

It is an anxiety that presents itself in the face of a real external danger. *Anxiety in the face of a real danger* is a feeling formed automatically and involuntarily by the individual who finds himself in a situation of psychological and biological helplessness, while the *neurotic anxiety* [*Neurotische Angst*] is a sign that serves precisely to avoid the repetition of this situation of danger that comes from within and no longer from without. Freud says,

> If so, it seems plausible to suppose that in neurotic anxiety the ego is making a similar attempt at flight from the demand by its libido, that it is treating this internal danger as though it were an external one.
>
> (Freud 1916–1917c: 405)

The neurotic anxiety, in this sense, instead of facing the external danger through physical escape, creates symptoms to try to defend itself from a situation imposed by its own libido, which cannot find outlets to satisfy itself.

According to *Group Psychology and the Analysis of the Ego* [*Massenpsychologie und Ich-analyse*], from 1921, *panic*, or *social anxiety*, arises in situations of disjunction of the relationship between individual and society. It happens when a social organization finds itself threatened with disappearance. This feeling is produced in the individuals who are in imminent social isolation, threatened by the removal of any relationship with others. The disintegration of the mass causes the formation of hostile feelings between individuals and the breaking of the ties that made union between them possible. "It is impossible to doubt that panic means the disintegration of a group; it involves the cessation of all the feelings of consideration which the members of the group otherwise show one another" (Freud 1921: 97), Freud says. *Panic* presupposes the loosening of affective bonds that keep the group cohesive, so that the individual, whose libidinal tendency is to come together in ever-larger collectivities, feels incomplete and unprotected.

In 1926, in the text *Inhibition, Symptom and Anxiety* [*Hemmung, Symptom und Angst*], Freud finally establishes his theory of anxiety, stating that every anxiety is a reaction to a dangerous situation, so that the ego is led to do something to avoid or to subtract itself from it. "[Anxiety] is therefore an affective reaction on the part of the ego to danger; and the danger which is being signalled in this way is the danger of castration" (Freud 1926: 126). Freud, then, wonders what the meanings of danger situations would be. The answer he offers is very clear: "A danger situation is a recognized, remembered, expected situation of helplessness" (Freud 1926: 166). The experience of helplessness represents the child's first separation from its mother so that anxiety appears as a sign of the repetition of this primordial separation. This first formation of anxiety will serve as a traumatic model for other traumatic situations. As soon as the ego recognizes a situation of danger analogous to separation from the mother, it gives signs of anxiety.

Freud identifies three factors involved in the formation of distress. The *phylogenetic* factor as a hereditary precipitate, inferred by the primitive conditions of the human being in its initial development. The *biological* factor, which refers to the long phase of helplessness and dependence of the newborn baby, is the origin of the first situations of danger. In this sense, anxiety arises as a sign of defence of the ego against threats of danger caused by its physical unpreparedness. And, finally, the *psychological* factor, which stems from the imperfections of the ego in defending itself from threats caused by the urgency of the drives. Norbert Elias's analysis of the court society allows us to add the *sociological* factor as a cause of anxiety, insofar as individuals had to guarantee their own existence by submitting themselves to the rules of etiquette and social coercion of this configuration. As Freud states,

> It is the absence of the mother that is now the danger; and as soon as that danger arises the infant gives the signal of anxiety, before the dreaded economic situation has set in. This change constitutes a first great step forward in the provision made by the infant for its self-preservation, and at the same time represents a transition from the automatic and involuntary fresh appearance of anxiety to the intentional reproduction of anxiety as a signal of danger.
>
> (Freud 1926: 138)

Little by little, the child grows up and becomes more independent. In the course of psychic maturation, some anxieties are abandoned because certain dangerous situations are no longer relevant. As the ego goes through repeated affective breaks throughout its constitution, it is being prepared for different experiences of loss and separation. When the individual is faced once again with a possible situation of helplessness, the anxiety signals a danger to avoid feeling threatened of losing the love of his object.

Continuing in *Inhibition, Symptom and Anxiety*, Freud describes the path of anxiety, from fear of loss of the *mother's* love, to fear of loss of the *superego's* love, to fear of loss of the *mass's* love, and to fear of *death*:

> The progress which the child makes in its development – its growing independence, the sharper division of its mental apparatus into several agencies, the advent of new needs – cannot fail to exert an influence upon the content of the danger situation. We have already traced the change of that content

> from loss of the mother as an object to castration. The next change is caused by the power of the super-ego. With the depersonalization of the parental agency from which castration was feared, the danger becomes less defined. Castration anxiety develops into moral anxiety – social anxiety – and it is not so easy now to know what the anxiety is about. The formula, "separation and expulsion from the horde", only applies to that later portion of the super-ego which has been formed on the basis of social prototypes, not to the nucleus of the super-ego, which corresponds to the introjected parental agency. Putting it more generally, what the ego regards as the danger and responds to with an anxiety-signal is that the super-ego should be angry with it or punish it or cease to love it. The final transformation which the fear of the super-ego undergoes is, it seems to me, the fear of death (or fear for life) which is a fear of the super-ego projected on to the powers of destiny.
>
> (Freud 1926: 139–140)

Anxiety then forms itself as a reaction to the lack of the desired object. In fact, says Freud, the anxiety resulting from the loss of the object happens because of the fear of losing the love one receives from it: "it is no longer a matter of feeling the want of, or actually losing the object itself, but of losing the object's love" (Freud 1926: 143). The anxiety of the first separation from the mother becomes anxiety in the face of the superego and, consequently, social anxiety. Anxiety, in this sense, no longer points to the threats of the loss of love of an external object, but to the threats of the loss of love of a psychic structure representing the parental insignia, the superego. The external danger becomes an internal danger. Given this scenario, in order to maintain the love and protection of the superego, the ego submits itself to the rigidity and severity of its rules. Freud, then, concludes that the ego is the actual seat of anxiety.

> But if we ask ourselves what it is that the ego fears from the super-ego, we cannot but think that the punishment threatened by the latter must be an extension of the punishment of castration. Just as the father has become depersonalized in the shape of the super-ego, so has the fear of castration at his hands become transformed into an undefined social or moral anxiety. But this anxiety is concealed. The ego escapes it by obediently carrying out the commands, precautions and penances that have been enjoined on it. If it is impeded in doing so, it is at once overtaken by an extremely distressing feeling of discomfort which may be regarded as an equivalent of anxiety and which the patients themselves liken to anxiety.
>
> (Freud 1926: 128)

To avoid anxiety, instead of running away as it would in the face of an external danger, the ego submits itself to the coercions of the superego in order to receive support and protection from it. The ego feels threatened with death in the same way as if it were at the mercy of objective forces. In this case, castration acts as an analogy of death, threatening to break the relationships of dependence that serve the conservation of the ego. Anxiety, in this way, shows itself as an emotion that arises not only when the ego is facing a situation of real danger, but also whenever there is risk of separation from its protective psychic structure.

Following Norbert Elias's goal of establishing a sociogenesis of the formation of unconscious psychic processes as proposed by Freud, we could affirm that social structures and psychic structures reflect certain operators of ancient social configurations, such as the light of a star that still propagates in the space even after its destruction. The new grammar of court societies inscribed disjunctions between the individual and society, between subject and object, and between nature and culture. A new condition of discontent has been formed by the detachment of individuals from their own bodies, from other individuals and from nature. What is part of the constitution of one is no longer related to what is part of the constitution of the other. We are alienated from the objects that cause our existence, alienated from our otherness, trapped in a nostalgia about a condition that is impossible to fulfil. And what should be more familiar to us becomes something strange to us, so that split in two in our very being we can no longer recognize each other.

In his analyses of court society, Norbert Elias explains that the nobility formed a specific *ethos* that endeavoured, at all costs, not to be threatened with losing the social recognition of honour and prestige that distinguished it from other classes. For this society of the *Ancien Régime*, the "maintenance of distance thus becomes a decisive motor or matrix of their behaviour. The value of this existence needs no justification for the people involved, above all no utilitarian explanation" (Elias 1969: 102). In the balance of tensions of the court configuration, any behaviour or emotion that produced an imbalance in the power games could put the individual in danger of being abandoned or excluded from the group of people at the same economic and social level. By breaking down the barriers that sustained the privileges of the upper social strata, the barriers that protected them from the pressure of the lower strata were broken down.

When recognition was refused by good society, the elements that gave meaning to the identity of individuals were lost, so that sometimes it was preferable to die rather than cease to be part of it. The individual, a social being par excellence, had his identity formed by the representation that others created of him: "the recognition of membership by others itself constitutes membership" (Elias 1969: 96). The risk and fear of being relegated to the margins of society represented, for courtiers, not only the loss of their human value, but also a threat of death, the end of their existence. In this sense, what was sought in the competition for prestige was, in the end, protection, love, and recognition by people on the same social level.

As we know, Norbert Elias' plans to achieve a university post were abruptly halted. On 30 January 1933, Adolf Hitler was appointed Chancellor of Germany. Less than two months later, a decree approved by the Nazi party removed all Jewish civil servants from their professional positions. Norbert Elias then was forced to abandon his desire to build an academic career and seek exile in another country. First, he lived in Switzerland, then in France, where he spent a period in which he failed in obtaining a university position, and finally in England, where he arrived in 1935. By that time, he had already finished his thesis on court society, a requirement to obtain the position of *Privatdozent* at the University of Frankfurt. But Elias was forced to put his thesis aside until it was published more than three decades after it was written, when he was already recognized by the academic community.

The studies on changes in everyday relationships continue with the research on etiquette manuals, in an attempt to understand how new *habitus*, new ways of controlling behaviour and emotions are formed. His gaze turned to apparently banal subjects, which were not part of the objects of interest of any researcher: the way to behaving at the table, to blowing one's nose, of spitting, of urinating and defecating, of washing and sleeping, as well as the sexual relationships and aggressiveness, but which determine the functioning of the psychic economy of individuals. These researches resulted in one of his best-known works, *The Civilizing Process*, published in 1939.

References

Elias, Norbert (1939) *The Civilizing Process*. Malden: Blackwell Publishing, 2013.

——— (1969) *The Court Society*. New York: Pantheon Books, 1983.

——— (1985/2000) "Norbert Elias ou la sociologie des continuités", in *Labyrinthe*, vol. 5, pp. 89–95.

——— (1987) *J'ai suivi mon propre chemin: un parcours dans le siècle*. Paris: Les Éditions Sociales, 2016.

——— (2014) "La sociologie... quand elle est bien faite. Entretien, 1984–1985", in *Actes de la recherche en sciences sociales*, vol. 205, n.5, p. 16, trans. by J. Durval and S. Noël. www.cairn.info/revue-actes-de-la-recherche-en-sciences-sociales-2014-5-page-4.htm

Freud, Sigmund (1916–1917c) "Anxiety", in *The Standard Edition of the Complete Psychological Works of Sigmund Freud – Introductory Lectures on Psycho-analysis (Part III)*, vol. XVI, ed. and trans. by J. Strachey. London: Hogarth Press, 1981.

——— (1921) "Group Psychology and the Analysis of the Ego", in *The Standard Edition of the Complete Psychological Works of Sigmund Freud – Beyond the Pleasure Principle, Group Psychology and Other Works (1920–1922)*, vol. XVIII, ed. and trans. by J. Strachey. London: Hogarth Press, 1981.

——— (1926) "Inhibition, Symptom and Anxiety", in *The Standard Edition of the Complete Psychological Works of Sigmund Freud – An Autobiographical Study, Inhibitions, Symptoms and Anxiety, The Question of Lay Analysis and Other Works (1925–1926)*, vol. XX, ed. and trans. by J. Strachey. London: The Hogarth Press, 1981.

——— (1930) "Civilization and Its Discontents", in *The Standard Edition of the Complete Psychological Works of Sigmund Freud – The Future of an Illusion, Civilization and its Discontents and Other Works (1927–1931)*, vol. XXI, ed. and trans. by J. Strachey. London: The Hogarth Press, 1981.

Joly, Marc (2012) *Devenir Norbert Elias*. Paris: Fayard.

2 The dynamics of the civilizing process

In April 1933, Norbert Elias left his hometown to begin a long life in exile. At first, he thought he would find opportunities in Switzerland for the teaching career he was just starting. Unsuccessfully he had to return to Germany, soon making his way to France. His time in Paris was also short. For a few months, between 1934 and 1935, he lived in Montparnasse *quartier*. The cafés in Paris helped him to meet some important people from the cultural and intellectual milieu. But the only one to invite him into his home was the philosopher and historian of sciences Alexandre Koyré, whose courses Elias attended at the *École Pratique des Hautes Études*. With no possibilities of work within French universities, Elias managed to publish his first article in sociology, entitled *The Kitsch style and the age of Kitsh* [*Kitschstil und Kitschzeitalter*].

With no money to support himself and already 38 years old, he ended setting up a wooden toy factory, specialized in wooden modelling, toys, and gift items, called *Les Ateliers Norbert* and located at number 34 rue de l'Abbé Groult in the 15th *arrondissement*. Together with two German-Jewish colleagues, the business did not last more than nine months, causing him to lose all the money he had invested. Against this background, Elias was invited to cross the English Channel and live in England. Elias reluctantly accepted the invitation because his English was not as fluent as the French language. With no prospects for his future and less and less money, his situation in the French capital, however, was already becoming unviable.

Arriving in England in 1935, Elias went to a committee for Jewish refugees, receiving a small amount of money so that he could continue his professional career. Thus, Elias began to frequent the British Museum library daily, working on a project that followed the methodology of long-term analysis of the formations of habits and behaviour patterns in different social settings, that led to the writing of his most notorious work, *The Civilizing Process* [*Über den Prozeß der Zivilisation: soziogenetische und psychogenetische Untersuchungen*]. Even with the forced departure from his country, Elias managed to maintain the creative force that, in Frankfurt, had motivated him to advance in the field of interdisciplinary research in an attempt to formalize the reciprocal transformations between social structures and psychic structures.

DOI: 10.4324/9781003378938-2

The image that Norbert Elias evokes of his parents and his childhood shows that he was a child extremely attached to them. "I knew that my father would do everything for me, and also my mother, too. If I was ill – and I was very frequently ill as a child – every care was taken; I felt completely protected" (Elias 1987: 14). The care his parents took throughout his life was fundamental. His mother's love and care, as well as the harmony of the couple, left a mark of security in his life. Elias continues: "I always think that the staying power I had later, when I wrote my books and no one took any notice of them, was due to the very great security that I enjoyed as a child" (Elias 1987: 14). In 1938, his parents went to London to visit him for the last time. Two years later his father died, and in 1941 his mother was sent to Auschwitz concentration camp, where she was murdered in one of the gas chambers. It was to his parents that Elias dedicated his most important work.

The publication of the first edition of *The Civilizing Process* only came about with the financial help Elias received from his father. Since Jews were no longer allowed access to their own bank accounts at the time, they were forced to go through the censorship of the Nazi authorities to have the money released. Sales of Elias's first book, however, were soon impeded by Nazi persecution of Jews. Just remember that six years earlier, Joseph Goebbels, Propaganda Minister of Nazi Germany, proclaimed a national act to clean up German literature, throwing into a huge public bonfire more than 25,000 works by authors such as Thomas Mann, Walter Benjamin, Bertolt Brecht, Robert Musil, Sigmund Freud, Albert Einstein, Karl Marx, and Heinrich Heine, among others. In 1939, Austria, Czechoslovakia, and Germany no longer allowed non-German books to be sold, especially works written by Jewish authors. This, however, did not prevent Elias's book from being distributed free of charge to magazines and newspapers. The second edition of the work, with an extended introduction, did not come out until 1969. This edition was responsible for bringing Elias out of oblivion.

2.1 The expansion of civilization

The investigations Norbert Elias undertook reiterated his effort to understand the reciprocity between changes in social structures and transformations in personality structures, seeking to overcome the dichotomy between the individual and society: "The psychogenesis of the adult make-up in civilized society cannot, therefore, be understood if considered independently of the sociogenesis of our civilization" (Elias 1939: xi), according to the preface of *The Civilizing Process*, written in 1936. At that point, however, it seemed necessary to begin to develop a general theory of the civilizing process capable of explaining how the transformations in social structures, during the long transition from feudal peoples to modern states, produced consequences in the psychic structures of individuals. In this sense, one can say that the sociological foundation of his research, starting from Max Weber's observation that the state is the monopoly of brute force, recovers the influence of Freud's psychoanalysis to reflect, with Marx's economic-philosophical thought, that societies are not only determined by the order of violence and the dominion of capital, but also by the pulsional economy of individuals.

Elias's project was to develop research against the claim of modern philosophy and sciences to understand their objects of analysis as if they were structures closed in themselves, autonomous and isolated from each other. In this sense, Elias attacked psychology, economics, sociology, and history, or rather all disciplines that thought that individuals and societies could be deciphered without considering them in a mutual and constant process of transformation. Thus, he presents the starting point of *The Civilizing Process*:

> If members of present-day Western civilized society were to find themselves suddenly transported into a past epoch of their own society, such as the medieval-feudal period, they would find there much that they esteem "uncivilized" in other societies today. Their reaction would scarcely differ from that produced in them at present by the behaviour of people in feudal societies outside the Western world. They would, depending on their situation and inclinations, be either attracted by the wilder, more unrestrained and adventurous life of the upper classes in this society, or repulsed by the "barbaric" customs, the squalor and coarseness that he encountered there. And whatever they understand by their own "civilization", they would at any rate feel quite unequivocally that society in this past period of Western history was nor "civilized" in the same sense and to the same degree as Western society today.
>
> (Elias 1939: ix)

A series of transformations in Western societies produced discomfort and repugnance towards certain attitudes towards public uses of bodily functions. Some habits were removed from everyday life to be classified as "barbarian" or "uncivilized". What could be the reasons that produced these changes in our behaviour and that transformed not only the way we relate to each other but also our own psychic economy? Starting from this question and by recovering the origins of the concept of civilization, Elias sets out to trace the clues of the civilizing process that transformed behaviour patterns over the centuries. That is, in the sociologist's words: "The question arises as to how and why Western society actually moved from one standard to the other, how it became 'civilized'" (Elias 1939: 51). Civilization, as we are accustomed to referring to it as the highest value of humanity has not come to us ready or finished. In this sense, what Elias seeks to clarify is how and why the structure of Western society changes at the same time as the behaviour patterns and psychic constitution of individuals change.

The methodology of Elias's research is close to that of psychoanalysis, insofar as Freud also sought to identify the meanings of unconscious formations in the psychopathology of everyday life. Elias, in his own way, turned to topics that were not evident to the eyes of any researcher because at first, they would not be worthy of scientific interest. He did not concern himself with great social revolutions, but with small changes in everyday life; he did not give prominence to sociological or philosophical theories, but to manuals of etiquette, books of literature and poetry; he did not set out to understand concepts and ideas, but to the habits of the everyday life of individuals.

On the one hand, Elias turned to the main Freudian concepts to support his thesis on the civilizing process. On the other hand, he did not shy away from criticizing psychoanalysis as a theory derived from the paradigms of modern science. One of the criticisms that the sociologist addresses to Sigmund Freud concerns the absence of historical processes in the elaboration of psychic instances. It is as if the psychoanalyst had thought of them as a ready-made structure, closed in itself, without having gone through a process of transformations over the centuries. Elias sought to understand the mutual interaction between psychic processes and changes in social structures, which does not allow us to consider the individual as a finished being, nor to think that there is a determined origin, a zero point of his constitution. There are no beginnings for Elias's processual sociology. Nor can we think that everything was there all along.

In the first volume of *The Civilizing Process*, Elias puts forward his critique of Freudian psychoanalysis:

> This, as has been mentioned, is clearly the state of affairs which Freud tried to express by concepts such as the "superego" and the "unconscious" or, as it is nor unfruitfully called in everyday speech, the "subconscious". But however it is expressed, the social code of conduct so imprints itself in one form or another on human beings that it becomes a constituent element of their individual selves. And this element, the superego, like the personality structure as a whole of individual people, necessarily changes constantly with the social code of behaviour and the structure of society. The pronounced division in the "ego" or consciousness characteristic of people in our phase of civilization, which finds expression in such terms as "superego" and "unconscious", corresponds to the specific split in the behaviour which civilized society demands of its members. It matches the degree of regulation and restraint imposed on the expression of drives and impulses. Tendencies in this direction may develop in any form of human society, even in those which we call "primitive". But the strength attained in societies such as ours by this differentiation and the form in which it appears are reflections of a particular historical development, the results of a civilizing process.
>
> (Elias 1939: 160)

For Elias, we cannot speak of superego as something static, universal and unchanging. On the contrary, we must consider that the psychic instances, as well as the drive economy, accompany the transformation of societies. The superego is social, the ego is social and the drives are social. This does not mean, however, that it is possible to determine their origins in some specific moment in history. There are changes in the use that each society makes of each one of these elements, that is, different societies vary on how they use the psychic economy. In this sense, Elias goes so far as to mark differences between a medieval catholic superego and a protestant superego, or between the superego of the courtly society and the bourgeois superego. In *The Civilizing Process*, he writes,

> One can see that in the course of human history, and again and again in that of each individual civilizing process, self-steering through ego and super-ego functions on the one hand and self-steering through drives on the other become more and more firmly *differentiated.* Hence it is only with the formation of conscious function less accessible to drives that the drive automatisms take on more and more that specific character which today is commonly diagnosed as "ahistoric", as a human characteristic throughout the ages which is purely natural, and independent of the developmental condition of human societies.
>
> (Elias 1939: 410)

The criticism that Elias sustains against Freud proceeds in the direction of thinking that psychoanalysis got stuck in theoretical reductionism when it failed to overcome the insurmountable wall of the relationship between individual and society. Freud, for the sociologist, forgot to consider the social and historical effects of the civilizing process in the formation of the conscious, the unconscious, and the drives. As if Freud had not thought of the individual from and within the processes of transformation of societies. In Elias's words,

> However, the human characteristic discovered by Freud in people of our own time and conceptualized by him as a strict division between unconscious and conscious mental functions, far from being part of humans' unchanged nature is a result of a long civilizing process in the course of which the wall of forgetfulness separating libidinal drives "consciousness" or "reflection" has become higher and more impermeable.
>
> (Elias 1939: 410)

In societies in which there is a strong use of physical violence and in which impulses are satisfied almost without restraint, individuals are bound to control their passions at the same time that they are vulnerable to the force of others' feelings. Over time, they learn to regulate themselves, building self-control mechanisms in the form of habits and behaviours that are repeated unconsciously. This is what Elias calls "softening of drives". On the other hand, the dangers that previously appeared explicitly in relationships with others are transferred, in the form of psychic conflicts, to the backstage of psychic life, to an "Other scene" [*eine andere Schauplatz*], using Freud's expression when referring to the place where psychic processes, beyond the stage of consciousness. The civilizing process, in this sense, reproduces as psychic conflicts the conflicts that previously presented themselves in social relations.

The Civilizing Process was originally published in two volumes, which, in turn, were divided into four main parts. To the first volume, whose subtitle is "Changes in the behaviour of the secular upper classes in the West" [*Wandlungen des Verhaltens in den weltlichen Oberschichten des Abendlandes*], Elias wrote to Walter Benjamin in a letter sent on 17 April 1938 to ask the German thinker for a review of his book: "Before us stands the more positive task of making the rules of the historical change in the psychical accessible to our understanding" (Elias 1938: 55). In the second volume, originally entitled "Changes in Society: Outline for a Theory of Civilization" [*Wandlungen der Gesellschaft: Entwurf zu einer Theorie der Zivilisation*], but published in English as "State Formation and Civilization", Elias explains to Benjamin what still needed to be done: "Then it remains for us to investigate, step by step, which social processes are the motors of this psychical change" (Elias 1938: 55). The second volume of *The Civilizing Process* is then devoted to formalizing a procedural theory of civilization.

In the first chapter of the first volume, "On the Sociogenesis of the Concepts of Civilization and Culture", Elias discusses the sociogenesis of the concepts of "culture" and "civilization" with reference to their usage in France and Germany from the 16th to the 18th centuries. With the different meanings of these terms, he seeks to understand how the behaviour and affective life of Western peoples was slowly transformed. The second chapter, "Civilization as a specific transformation of Human Behaviour" focuses on the civilizing psychic process by analyzing the habits and behaviour, etiquette, and social norms of societies in transition from the medieval period to modern times. With numerous examples taken from textbooks, historical documents, and literature, we see how the process of internalization of external coercions has been taking place in the form of psychic mechanisms of self-control and the consequent production of affections such as shame and fear.

Norbert Elias's most notorious book begins by investigating national *self-images* through the historical situations, whose atmosphere surrounding the formation of the terms *civilité* and *civilisation* in French, and the antithesis between *Kultur* and *Zivilisation* in German. These words carry the repressions operated by the civilizing process in meanings that the speaker himself does not know of their existence, for, forgotten by the linguistic community, they have been silently transmitted and reproduced through successive generations:

> The social process of their genesis may be long forgotten. One generation hands them on to another without being aware of the process as a whole, and the concepts live as long as this crystallization of past experiences and situations retains an existential value, a function in the actual being of society – that is, as long as succeeding, generations can hear their own experiences in the meaning of the words.
>
> (Elias 1939: 08)

Thus, Elias places himself as a researcher involved in the analysis of words that identify the way societies and individuals construct their own images and attribute values to themselves. The meanings that have been repressed and are therefore unknown to the speakers themselves, but remain strong and active through the "crystallization of the past embodied in words" (Elias 1939: 09). The French use of the term *civilisation* turned out to be a parameter for evaluating the conditions of a certain society in relation to another. *Civilisation* expresses the consciousness of a society, which allows it to measure itself as superior or inferior to any other. For both the English and the French, the concept of civilization referred to material productions, technological level, attitudes and behaviour, religious ideas, bodily cleanliness, etc. In other words, civilization encompassed everything that indicated the progress of the West and of humanity and thereby represented levels of superiority in relation to other societies.

The creation of an opposition with the "simple man" – and its maximum expression in the figure of the *bon sauvage*, according to the mythology developed by philosopher Jean-Jacques Rousseau (1762) – indicated that the civilizing process had managed to reach a higher degree in human evolution. The *homme civilisé* ended up marking the ideal of all the "good societies" of this period, determining the characteristics of the cultured and polished man. He was the reference point with which all nations identified themselves, would like to be and to see reproduced so that

> this concept expresses the self-consciousness of the West. One could even say: the national consciousness. It sums up everything in which Western society of the last two or three centuries believes itself superior to earlier societies or "more primitive" contemporary ones.
>
> (Elias 1939: 5)

Civilization portrayed the *self-image* of the European upper class over the centuries and levelled its members as superiors relative to individuals of other nationalities. However, the term "civilization" carried differences in each country's uses of it to construct a national *self-image*. For the English and French, speaking in terms of civilization, qualifying something as civilized or barbarian, served not only to establish limits of superiority but also to justify the ideologies of exploration and colonization movements, keeping national identity sovereign and borders secure in the logic of colonizing projects. A Western country of the 18th century considered itself more civilized than an indigenous tribe of the same century, thus justifying the self-congratulatory need to universalize its own characteristics over other societies considered inferior by themselves.

When Elias says that the term civilization serves to describe "the level of its technology, the nature of its manners, the development of its scientific knowledge or view of the world, and much more" (Elias 1939: 5), he emphasizes pronouns that indicate the possession of something that makes a society distinct and superior to others. A civilized people possess more, is more complex, is more cohesive and more balanced. And this always leads to a position of differentiation and power in relation to another uncivilized or barbarian people, who possess less, is less peaceful, less cohesive and less stable. This is a concept that overvalues a national identity and, as an effect of comparisons, reinforces the colonizing tendency of domination. Elias continues,

> Whereas the concept of civilization has the function of giving expression to the continuously expansionist tendency of colonizing groups, the concept of *Kultur* mirrors the self-consciousness of a nation which had constantly to seek out and constitute its boundaries anew, in a political as well as a spiritual sense.
>
> (Elias 1939: 7)

Until the 19th century, civilization could be considered by intellectuals and people of high social class, a complete and finished process. As a standard of measure, the idea of civilization formed a common identity among individuals belonging to the same nation, but also served as a model whose reference narcissistically allowed the colonization and transformation of any other society according to its own model. In Elias's words: "To the upper and middle classes of their own society, civilization appeared as a firm possession. They wished above all to disseminate it, and at most to develop it within the framework of the standard already reached" (Elias 1939: 88–89). If civilization represents the intrinsic value of a society, delimiting national differences and projecting identities among all, it was in the concept of *Kultur* that the German people found an expression to give special emphasis to their self-consciousness. As Elias points out, "The word through which Germans interpret themselves, which more than any other expresses their pride in their own achievements and their own being, is *Kultur*" (Elias 1939: 6). For all Germans who were not part of the nobility, the word *Zivilisation* was in the background, referring to the superficiality of appearances. The concept *Kultur*, on the other hand, referred to finished products such as works of art, books, religious and philosophical systems as forms of expression of the uniqueness of a people.

The term *Kultur* helps to answer the question, "What really is our identity?" (Elias 1939: 7). It gets to the point of what determines that structure, without needing to compare itself with another to establish its own boundaries. In answering the question "what is really German?" – which, according to Elias, has long since ceased to be answered by French and English nations – lies the peculiar element of *Kultur*, which searches in the essence of a people's identity for the fundamental traits of its constitution. In the German context, the middle class was formed by an intellectual elite belonging to the bourgeoisie, distant from the circles of the nobility and holder of the bureaucratic power of administration of public institutions. The bourgeoisie, then, inscribed the *Kultur* of its elite in the formation of the individual through literature, philosophy and the sciences, while the aristocracy turned to the customs of *Zivilisation*, identified with the national ideals of the French nobility as the centre of *civilisation*. From this social contrast arose the distinction between *Zivilisation* and *Kultur*, representing the differences between a noble class that spoke French, was concerned with good society, the control of feelings by reason, and decided on politics, and a bourgeois intelligentsia, which spoke German, turned to the depth of feelings, the development of personality, intellectual training, and had no influence on politics.

In the conflict of words, social conflicts are manifested: "the doors below must remain shut. Those above must open" (Elias 1939: 18). The walls between one class and another in Germany remained very high, making it very difficult to move into more privileged social strata. Thus, the aristocratic models of the German court and the bourgeois values remained separated for a long time. The social antithesis that emerges from the analysis of the terms *Zivilisation* and *Kultur*, as it occurred in the German context, comes to develop in the form of a national antithesis. What was once a conflict between social classes takes on forms to represent the national *self-image*, responding to the defining traits of what is German, which in turn come to form the personality of German individuals.

The second part of the first volume of *The Civilizing Process* deals with the history of the transformation of customs in relation to the sociogenesis of the concept of *civilisation* in France. In this case, unlike Germany, the distance between the bourgeois *intelligentsia* and courtly society was not so unbridgeable. By the 18th century, bourgeois customs had already absorbed the etiquette of the court aristocracy, forming a more unitary and cohesive national *self-image* than the German case, since the French bourgeoisie was closer to the court, participating in political activities and the administration of the state.

The concept of civilization, as Elias indicates, first appears in the French language with the writer Victor Riquetti de Mirabeau (1715–1789), author of works such as *L'ami des hommes ou Traité de la population*, written in 1757. In the same vein as Elias, Émile Benveniste, when dealing with the term civilization in his book *Problems in General Linguistics* (1966), also recognizes in the Marquis de Mirabeau the first French use of the term civilisation. In English language, the term civilization appears for the first time, according to Benveniste, in *An Essay on the History of Civil Society*, by the professor of moral philosophy Adam Ferguson, written in Edinburgh in 1767. According to Benveniste's investigations, there is nothing to indicate that the Scottish writer was inspired by Mirabeau's literature, so that the question remains open as to whether the term civilization was originally coined in France and England, independently of each other, or whether it is only the French language that invented this vocabulary for modern Europe.

Both Norbert Elias and Benveniste have highlighted the following fragment from a work by Mirabeau, written in 1768, called *L'ami des femmes ou Traité de la civilisation*, but which was never published. Located in the *Archives Nationales* in Paris and containing five and a half pages of introduction and ten pages of argument, it reads,

> I admire in this respect how our views of research are wrong in every respect about what we hold to be civilization. If I were to ask most of you what you think civilization consists of, I would be told, civilization is the softening of morals, urbanity, politeness, and the spread of knowledge in such a way that manners are observed and that they take the place of laws of detail; all this presents to me only the mask of virtue and not its face, and civilization does nothing for society if it does not give it the substance and form of virtue.
>
> (Mirabeau *quoted* Benveniste 1966: 291)

Mirabeau's use of the term civilization is close to what was hitherto called *police*, that is, an act of policing that leads individuals to observe more spontaneously their behaviours according to the rules of convenience in order to urbanize their social customs. Norbert Elias's reading of this same quote by Mirabeau also points to a term that represents the ideal of the court aristocracy, to which everyone would like to align themselves, and which becomes a virtue a general characteristic of European society. A concept used by the nobility to universalize the qualities of their behaviours. Civilized was an individual *civilisé*, *poli* or *policé*, whose qualities and refinements of their ways of behaving were made into standards for socially inferior individuals, while expanding to the other European courts.

Thus, civilization carries a teleological meaning, a process with a direction towards achieving the standards of court society, through education, the formation of a rationality of etiquette and manners, the pacification of drives, and moral self-control. Civilization is the mark of the evolution of civilized individual, capable of integrating the highest social echelons, transmitting and colonizing other individuals and other nations in order to reproduce in them his complete and finalized state. All this, as Norbert Elias relates, was happening "In the name of the Cross, and later in that of civilization. Western society waged, during the Middle Ages, its wars of colonization and expansion" (Elias 1939: 47), preserving in its banner the mottos of Christianity and the Crusades of the medieval knights. But civilization forgot its process. It has repressed its contradictions and left on the surface the appearances, the evolutions, the hegemonies and power dominations, reproducing the habitus of the social class and the nation it represents.

Just as Freud (1986: 207)[1] pointed out to his friend Wilhelm Fliess, in the *Letter 52*, the repression is a psychic operation that fails to translate certain psychic contents from previous times to more current phases, leaving remnants in the memory that survive the passage of time. "Thus an anachronism persists: in a particular province, *fueros* are still in force; we are in the presence of 'survivals'" (Freud 1986: 208), Freud states, referring to the preservation of old Spanish laws in certain provinces that served to protect centuries-old privileges of those regions. In the same way, Elias concludes regarding the civilizing process: "Of the whole preceding process of civilization nothing remained in their consciousness except a vague residue" (Elias 1939: 43). It is not, however, residues that persists without effect for society and for individuals. In the same way that the repressed returns distorted as formations of the unconscious, determining symptoms and forms of psychic suffering in individuals, the process of civilization produces residues that are not completely erased in the course of social transformations, but remain preserved as habits, customs, and affections. Repetitions of social structures, finally, are analogous to repetitions of the unconscious.

2.2 The etiquette and the repression of drives

The ways of behaving at the table, the attitude toward bodily functions, the nose-blowing, the spitting, the urination and the defecation in public, the behaviours in the bedroom, such as the ways of sleeping and sexual relations, the exposure of the naked body in public spaces, the expressions of aggressiveness. In the formation of court societies, these and other behaviours were civilized to create a new etiquette. It was through etiquette manuals that Norbert Elias was able to demonstrate the effects of the civilizing process on the pulsional economy of individuals. In a sociological search for lost time, Elias investigated the changes among habits and customs that were no longer socially accepted. Let see some examples given by Elias in *The Civilizing Process*.

The poem, *Hofzucht*, written by Tannhäuser in the 13th century and intended exclusively for the upper class and court knights, featured rules such as: "If a man snorts like a seal when he eats, as some people do, and smacks his chops like a Bavarian yokel, he has given up all good breeding" (Tannhäuser *quoted* Elias 1939: 56). In *Courtesies*, by Bonvicino della Riva, an Italian table guide of the 13th century, Elias draws the following recommendation: "Do not slurp with your mouth when eating from a spoon. This is a bestial habit" (Bonvicino della Riva *quoted* Elias 1939: 73). Caxton's *The Book of Curtesye*, from the late 15th century, was a poem explaining the changes in social habits:

> Thingis whilom used ben now leyd a syde
> And newe feeris, dayly ben contreuide
> Mennys actes can in no plyce abyde
> They be changeable ande ofte meuide
> Thingis somtyme alowed is now repreuid
> And after this shal thinges up aryse
> That men sec now but at lytyl pryse.
> (Caxton *quoted* Elias 1939: 70–71)

The Babee's Book: Medieval Manners for the Young, a short treatise from the 14th century, regulated the habit of eating as follows: "If a man wipes his nose on his hand at table because he knows no bether, then he is a fool, believe me" (Furnivall *quoted* Elias 1939: 75). The civilizing process inscribes social controls that remove behaviours, desires, and emotions considered socially inadequate from the public sphere to place them in the private life of individuals. Many other examples from European court literature allowed us to understand how the civilizing process led to the inscription of certain habits in individuals, transforming external coercions into self-coercions.

Antoine de Courtin's 1672 book *Nouveau traité de civilité*, written when court society was already more consolidated, taught certain habits of civility to well-born young men who did not attend court. In it, you can find phrases like: "*Formerly, for example, it was permitted to split on the ground before people of rank, and was sufficient to put one's foot on the sputum. Today that is an indencency*" (Courtin *quoted* Elias 1939: 130). The 1702 book *Les règles de la bienséance et de la civilité chrétienne*, by Jean-Baptiste de La Salle, disseminated courtly models throughout the bourgeoisie, with rules such as: "*It is very impolite to emit wind from your body when in company. either from above or from below; even if it is done without noise*" (La Salle *quoted* Elias 1939: 112); "As far as natural needs are concerned, it is proper (even for children) to satisfy them only where one cannot be seen" (La Salle *quoted* Elias 1939: 113); or "It is very impolite to keep poking your finger into your nostrils, and still more insupportable to put what you have pulled from your nose into your mouth" (La Salle *quoted* Elias 1939: 125).

The nakedness of the body should be hidden from other people's eyes. Body odours should be concealed. Bodily excretions were to be made in specific places and away from everyone. The tendency among people to watch each other increased, so that the gaze was given a regulatory function for anything that escaped the norm. Norbert Elias consulted many other manuals on education to show how the transition from one social class to another gradually shaped habits and regulated affections, changing their personalities by inscribing automatic forms of self-control that served to segregate individuals.

It was in the work of Erasmus of Rotterdam where Elias found the most expressive example of how the transformations in the psychic structures of individuals were processed by the incorporation of social habits. Especially in the book *On Civility in Children* [*De civilitate morum puerilium*], written in 1530, Elias identified an important use of the concept of *civilité* to refer to "the behaviour of people in society – above all, but not solely, 'outward bodily propriety'" (Elias 1939: 48). From the term *civilitas*, other words were derived: *civilité* in French, *civility* in English, *civilità* in Italian, and *Zivilität* in German. The term *courtoise*, used with a sense of courtesy by the chivalry-feudal, was left aside to introduce the concept of *civilité* as a reference to the manners of the new aristocracies of the absolutist courts. Later, as the bourgeoisie approached the courtly nobility of France, the concept of *civilité* lost force to the use of the new term *civilisation*, reflecting the self-consciousness of a new absolutist nation that was emerging.

Considered the first treatise on moral and practical education for children, recording rules of conduct transmitted orally over generations and humanist in its purpose of establishing general human norms, the work *On Civility in Children*, by Rotterdam, delineates the patterns of behaviour that were no longer part of our social relationship and could therefore be called "barbarians" as opposed to those that remained and were referred to as "civilized". Dedicated to a noble boy, son of a prince, this essay served to educate conduct in social life situations, but it still carried with it the marks of an earlier time, situating itself between feudal culture and modern tradition, forming customs and rules of a new courtly society that was being constituted.

Norbert Elias' research on Erasmus's treatise gave clues to the times when the civilizing process was displacing external coercion towards forms of self-control. Times when it began to be a greater policing of behaviour and emotions, increasing the pressure that people exerted on each other. In a long-term process, that is to say: "Not abruptly but very gradually the code of behaviour became stricter and the degree of consideration expected of others became greater" (Elias 1939: 69). Thus, gradually, what should no longer be exposed in public was being repressed as unspoken and unthought content: violence, aggressiveness, drives, desires, and sexuality. As an effect of this repressing, specific affections in the relations between individuals were being formed: shame, fear, anxiety, disgust, and guilt. While the behaviours were being transformed in the upper class of the court, emotions were also being modified and, little by little, disseminated throughout society. The consequences of the internalization process were pacification and greater predictability of social ties. Individuals no longer needed to be alerted all the time to defend themselves from any type of attack that could come unexpectedly from any other person because society itself began to regulate everyone's behaviour.

Forgetfulness is an important mechanism of the civilizing process. Current civilization has forgotten that it is not ready or finished and that it develops in a long-lasting process that has no end. Individuals have forgotten that habits and customs are neither natural nor inherent, but form a *second nature* that results from the internalization of social rules. Individuals do not know why they do what they do or why they say what they say. They do and say it because it seems natural to them, since from childhood they are taught to behave in this way and they have always seen others acting in the same way. Habits become the automatisms of repetition, the mark of society on each person's being, and end up being transmitted between generations in an unconscious process in the form of acquired social knowledge. Its crystallization marks experiences and situations with existential values, so that the individual is only able to identify his existence by the meaning of his habits.

With this, says Elias,

> The social standard to which the individual was first made to conform from outside by external restraint is finally reproduced more or less smoothly within him or her, through a self-restraint which operates to a certain degree even against his or her conscious wishes.
>
> (Elias 1939: 109).

As patterns of repetition according to the internal automatism of each one, the imprint of society on the individual appears in the form of the superego. The conflicts that presented themselves outside individuals are not erased, but internalized and forgotten. The Freudian formulation that no memory is lost because the mnemic materials that are conserved in the unconscious reappear in the form of a symptom, translates Elias's hypothesis that certain patterns of behaviour, built up as social habits are repetitions whose origins are forgotten and intentions are ignored.

The human being cannot be thought of except through the relationship of interdependence with others, as well as his behaviours and emotions are not natural reflexes, but result from a learning process that stems from the fact that he is included in a society. Habits are the result of distinction between social classes, but they appear as if they have always existed. If the concept of interdependence emerges as a central element in Eliasian theory and through it is possible to understand how and why individuals establish ties with each other, the movement of exclusion from interpersonal relationships is a counterpart that accompanies by the same force and intensity, that is, in the civilizing process the movements of belonging also produce movements of exclusion. Interdependence and the instruments of civilization assume a double aspect, for while that they lead to inclusion in social groups through the renunciation of the satisfaction of drives they also "they always also serve as a weapon against social inferiors, a means of distinction. Handkerchief, fork, plates and all related implements were at first luxury articles with a particular social prestige value" (Elias 1939: 128), states Elias. Those who do not participate in the same civilizing process and do not reproduce the same habits are destined to be excluded as outsiders.

The Civilizing Process is one of Elias's works, where psychoanalysis is most evident, to the extent that it was to Sigmund Freud that the sociologist one of the first printed copy. As a thank-you reply, Elias received a postcard that was kept until the end of his life. In a note, the sociologist insists on the importance of Freud for his thought, without, however, failing to mention the existence of differences between them:

> In this connection it scarcely needs to be said, but is perhaps worth emphasizing explicitly, how much this study owes to the discoveries of Freud and the psychoanalytical school. The connections are obvious to anyone acquainted with psychoanalytical writings, and it did not seem necessary to point them our in particular instances, especially because this could not have been done without lengthy qualifications.
>
> (Elias 1939: 527)

Along the civilizing process, the repressing of impulses, affections, and behaviours transfers to the sphere of intimacy all those relations among people crossed by the four main sources of the drive: the look, the voice, the mouth, the ears, as Freud determined in 1915, in the study *Instincts and their Vicissitudes* [*Trieb und Triebschicksale*]. In this sense, considering the conflict between drives and social demands, psychoanalysis appears, in the words of Elias, "psychological theories of modern times" (Elias 1939: 127). More and more divisions are being set up that enclose the individual in an isolated compartment, establishing for him antinomies with his own body, with the external world, with other people.

With the division between intimate and collective life, placing what is allowed to be publicly performed and what should be restricted to private life, social prohibitions start to reproduce themselves in individuals in the form of self-control over the drives, establishing as a result a new psychic economy. What was once an object of desire can no longer be attained; what before aroused pleasure now provokes disgust; what once caused hatred is pacified for the common good. In a line of reasoning very close to that of psychoanalysis, according to which desire is the result of its own interdiction, Elias writes: "It is highly characteristic of civilized people that they are denied by socially instilled self-controls from spontaneously touching what they desire, love or hate" (Elias 1939: 170). As a consequence of the internalization of social coercion, some behaviours that are not socially acceptable become taboo when performed with others. A psychic conflict is generated which transfers the satisfactions of the drives behind the curtains of consciousness.

Among other objectives, Elias tries to historicize the personality structure through the effects of the civilizing process. The drives, as well as the psychic instances – the id, the ego and the superego – are effects of historical and social processes, varying according to time, social code and society organization. The last chapter of the second part of *The Civilizing Process*, concerning the changes in aggressiveness in the passage from feudal life to the urban life of the court, is essential for understanding the effects of changes in social structures on personality structures. At this point, Elias can articulate the empirical investigations of the first volume of *The Civilizing Process* with the theoretical formulations of the second volume of the work.

When Elias proposes to identify the social processes behind the formation of the psychic structure, he turns against a natural and universal conception of the human condition. To affirm that the drives result from the different ties that organize societies does not mean to say that the psychic apparatus, as Freud presented us, was formed in a certain society or in a certain historical period. The impulses, the libido, the superego are formations which are structured in different ways according to the different social configurations, but the tendency of this process is the internalization of the external forms of self-coercion in psychic instances of self-regulation of behaviours. In this sense, the conflict zone passed from the outside to the inside of the individual. In the same way that external fears were appeased and social environments became more pacified, for example, the internal fears and the production of particular symptoms and affections grew. It was up to the individual to resolve within himself the conflicts and tensions, which before were directed at the relationship with others.

The introduction of the use of cutlery at the table, for example, was not due to the need to be more careful with the transmission of disease or for education to one's neighbour, but to the fact that there was a growing dependence on the upper classes, as the driving force of civilization. The relationship with objects is linked to the habits assumed by a certain social class, producing effects on the psychic economy, therefore, on the drives and affections. The use of the fork, around the 17th century, led people to abandon the habit of eating with the hands by civilized behaviour. Habits, then, which are apparently considered natural, were forged little by little as an effect of social and pulsional transformations that took place over the centuries.

When the social grammar is transformed, the psychic economy is also transformed. Aggressiveness, according to Elias, reduces in function of certain social characteristics: the division of functions, the degree of dependence of individuals among themselves and the formation of self-control mechanisms. This, however, does not mean that it can be eliminated during the civilizing process: "It is as much transformed, 'refined', 'civilized', as all the other forms of pleasure" so that "it is only in dreams or in isolated outbursts that account for as pathological that something of its immediate and unregulated force appears" (Elias 1939: 161–162). The drives are part of the emotional structure of the individual, but their dynamics suffer the movements of the social grammar in which the individual is inserted.

Thus, Elias develops the idea that in a society with a weaker central power there are not many elements that act to contain aggressiveness. When the central power is strong, individuals are coerced into living in peace with each other, increasing the degree of identification between them and making the legality of violence available to the representatives of this power. The changing level of aggressiveness in a society results from social and historical transformations. For example, in warrior societies looting, robbery and murder were commonplace and were part of the social habits. Individuals had always to be on the alert for any unexpected reaction from people. If the future, for them, was unpredictable, the attitude they assumed in the face of death was not to fear it, as we do nowadays because death showed itself as an inescapable way out.[2] Elias states:

> Outbursts of cruelty did not exclude one from social life. They were not outlawed. The pleasure in killing and torturing others was great, and it was a socially permitted pleasure. To a certain extent, the social structure even pushed its members in this direction, making it seem necessary and practically advantageous to behave in this way.
>
> (Elias 1939: 163)

A society that had a looser social control also had a greater malleability in the changes of affections. In medieval societies, there was no central power that operated as a control on the discharge of emotions and physical attacks between people, so that emotional attitudes were marked by intensity, oscillation, and immediacy. To the spontaneity of aggressive acts corresponded the explosion of joy and the search for pleasures. The spontaneity of affective expressions in children, produced by the lack of instances of self-regulation, approximates the outbursts of affections in societies that do not possess external instances of violence control, as Elias describes:

> The drives, the emotions were vented more freely, more directly, more openly than later. It is only to us, in whom everything is more subdued, moderate and calculated, and in whom social taboos are built much more deeply into the fabric of our drive-economy as self-restraints, that the unveiled intensity of this piety, belligerence or cruelty appears to be contradictory... And because emotions were here expressed in a manner that in our own world is generally observed only in children, we call these expressions and forms of behaviour "childish".
>
> (Elias 1939: 168–169)

With the centralization of life in court societies and in increasingly concentrated urban spaces, new mechanisms for regulating behaviour and emotions were required new forms of circulation of the psychic economy. People were no longer as free as were the knights or the lords of the castles. They began to live at court and to be subject to the gaze of others. They have to behave according to strict rules and in conformity with their social positions. They have to model their gestures and affections, language and manner of speaking to suit the best way of dealing with other people.

Elias wrote *The Civilizing Process* in exile, fleeing from a political system that was beginning to persecute and exterminate certain individuals. How can we think of civilization and its process in the face of one of the greatest barbarities of humanity? How to think of civilization in the face of such violence? Eliasian sociology was often read as a form of praise of Western European societies and its author considered an evolutionist thinker, unable to deal with what was showing itself in his own eyes. The proposal of this book is to present a reading of Elias's work which goes against the criticism that fails to understand it as a way of responding to the problem of violence and the eruption of barbarism, that which produces ruptures in social structures and in personality structures. The search for the foundations of Sigmund Freud's psychoanalytic theory in the thought of Norbert Elias helps to bring important elements to show that the destinies of the drive's repression do not allow the process of formation of civilizations to happen without the production of unease, building invisible walls between individuals, their own bodies and the other individuals who compose societies.

2.3 A new grammar of the court society

Throughout the two volumes of *The Civilizing Process*, Norbert Elias deals with the transformations of social processes that set in motion transformations in psychic structures. In the third part of his *Magnum Opus*, "Feudalization and State Formation", we find an extensive analysis of the long period spanning the 11th and 17th centuries, from which the courts began to accumulate military and economic power, consolidating themselves as models that formed social codes, customs and tastes. The fourth and last part, "Synopsis: Toward a Theory of Civilizing Processes", takes up again the work, proposing a theory on civilizing processes to think about the links and relations between social processes and psychic processes so that, finally, "some light is shed on the formation of the 'super-ego' and on the relation of the conscious and unconscious impulses in the psyche of civilized people" (Elias 1939: xiii). Elias's analyses, however, could not disregard the mutual interactions between changes in social structures, which led to the transition from feudal societies to absolutist states, and changes in psychic structures, especially the strengthening of superego controls.

In the period analyzed by Elias, the figure of the king was beginning to establish itself as an absolute power. The moment people left life in the countryside or in small, decentralized courts attracted to life within urban centres and in large court societies, the domains of monarchical institutions and the centralization of powers in the hands of a single individual increased. The *centrifugal forces* that acted by fragmenting kingdoms into small courts and principalities reduced to make way for *centripetal forces*, which turned towards a single gravitational centre, the court society, establishing a communicating vessels model between the absolutist societies that encompassed much of Western Europe.

Members of European court societies spoke the same language, read the same books, had the same habits and tastes. The French court, whose apogee reached during the reign of Louis XIV, was the main reference for other court societies. Located in Versailles, it inspired standards of behaviour that served to watch over and controlled all those around it, while distinguishing social classes between those who belonged to the court and those who did not. In Germany, for example, the aristocracy wrote and spoke in French as a way of approximating to the customs of the French court. In the book *The Last Days of Immanuel Kant*, written by Thomas de Quincey from the work of Ehrgott Wasianski, disciple and friend of the German philosopher, we see Kant's transgression by writing directly in German:

> For it was a significant fact – significant of that great revolution in conscious dignity which, early in the eighteenth century, had begun to dawn upon the German race – that Leibnitz, the forerunner of Kant, holding the same station in philosophy for the fifty years between 1666 and 1716, which Kant held for the fifty years between 1750 and 1800, wrote chiefly in French; and, if at any time not in French, then in Latin; whereas Kant wrote almost exclusively in German. And why? Simply because all the sovereign princes in Germany, that found nothing amiss in German dollars and crowns, drew their little Aulic machineries in so servile a spirit of mimicry from France, that the very breath of their nostrils was the foul, heated atmosphere of Versailles, "laid on" (as our water companies say) at second-hand for German use.
>
> (De Quincey 1827: 100)

Through language, habits and customs, etiquette, ceremonial rites, ways of regulating behaviour and affections, societies were little by little distinguishing themselves and building their own identities. All this amid strong pressure between social classes. On the one hand, the upper classes exerted a fascination over the lower classes. At the same time, the nobles were regulated by the constant threat of being excluded from the *grand monde* and thrown into the large group of outsiders. One had to know how to choose one's words and gestures carefully in order not to run the risk of being excluded from life in society. Elias states

> That the gradual formation of this absolutist-courtly society was accompanied by a transformation of the drive-economy and conduct of the upper class in the direction of "civilization", has been shown by a series of examples. It has also been indicated how closely this increased restraint and regulation of elementary urges is bound up with increased social constraint, the growing dependence of the nobility on the central lord, the king or prince.
>
> (Elias 1939: 191)

It was not by mere chance, therefore, that the configuration of absolutist states was accompanied by the containment and moderation of passions. The increased differentiation between individuals, the complexification of their social functions, the growing dependence that was established between them, all these changes meant that each person was compelled to control their behaviour and affective reactions in order to live in a more stable and more predictable way. Thus, a new psychic economy was being formed in increasingly "civilized" courts. Elias continues,

> The civilizing of conduct and the corresponding transformation of the structure of mental and emotional life cannot be understood without tracing the process of state-formation, and within it the advancing centralization of society which first found particularly visible expression in the absolutist form of rule.
>
> (Elias 1939: 191)

Configured in a new social grammar, the monarchic state ended up imposing controls and coercions on individuals for the maintenance of a more stable, more balanced and more cohesive life. Little by little, habits have been built up as models of self-control, reorganizing the personality structure in a new drive economy. Competition between different social classes searching for honour, power and prestige instituted a rational calculus that came to regulate one's intentions and actions, so that "the shaping of the affections, the structure of drives and consciousness, in short, the whole social structure of personality and people's social attitudes necessarily change at the same time", says Elias (1939: 268).

Throughout the second volume of *The Civilizing Process*, Norbert Elias develops the thesis that the formation of modern states occurred from the development of a double monopoly. The *economic monopoly* focused on the collection of taxes and charges for services and products that increasingly circulated between territories, and the *monopoly of violence*, which, based on Max Weber's definition in *Politics as a Vocation* [*Politik als Beruf*], 1919, where he says, "we must say that the state is the form of a human community that (successfully) lays claim to the *monopoly of the legitimate physical violence* within a particular territory – and this idea of 'territory' is an essential defining feature" (Weber 1919: 33 – emphasis in original), legitimized the Royal Army to use force and power to pacify relations between people. As the management of power developed in the hands of a single individual, the prince or king, a centralizing administration came to take shape in the form of nation-states then, says Elias, "It is only with the emergence of this continuing monopoly of the central authority and this specialized apparatus for ruling that dominions take on the character of 'states'" (Elias 1939: 191).

State control over violence leads to the need for self-regulation that subjects the individual to the coercive laws determined by society, which leads to the process of self-regulation. At the same time, the economic control that presents itself in the logic of free competition imposes threats aimed at opening or closing access to places of prestige and privilege, regulating the status of each social class. In this logic, Elias states,

> Whoever does not rise, falls back. Victory, therefore, means in the first place – whether this is intended or not – dominance over one's closest rivals and their reduction to a position of dependence. The gain of one is here necessarily the other's loss, whether in terms of land, military capacity, money or any other resource of social power.
>
> (Elias 1939: 305)

This struggle endangers not only the social position of individuals, leading the excluded to social decay, but, above all, endangering his very existence.

The grammar of the court society is based on a balance of tensions between the different social classes, as in a game of tug-of-war, in which two sides pull the rope as hard as they can without either player being able to strike a final blow against the other and fall apart with everything. In the formation of court societies, the nobility had to contend mainly with the competitions imposed by the bourgeois groups, which grew with the commercial movements of the 16th century. The nobility and the bourgeoisie became increasingly dependent on each other, in a relationship marked by a game of interests in which the aim of those below was to achieve the same conditions of privilege.

The upper and lower classes could not force the fragile balance of tensions in order not to lose the guarantees of acquired opportunities, but neither could they avoid conflict, insofar as any gain by the other was considered a threat to their own social position. "Accordingly, there was on the one hand no lack of courteous and even friendly relationships between members of the different groups" while Elias continues further, "each feared the other; each observed the other's steps with constant if concealed mistrust" (Elias 1939: 326). Thus, social coercions and the fascination of economic privileges of the upper classes doubly alienated individuals in a life directed by the desire to achieve better conditions.

Elias begins the synopsis of *The Civilizing Process* from the social transformations that made possible the change of social control into self-control, so that certain behaviours and emotions were excluded from social life to the unconscious backstage of psychic life. To explain how the civilizing process modified the psychic economy of individuals, Elias compares the same scene taking place in two different eras. The way individuals travel the streets and roads shows the different levels of integration with society. First, we should visualize how it was a society formed by people used to daily fights and wars, in contact with the most varied types of personalities and, therefore, having to be alert to the most unpredictable situations.

> With few exceptions, there is very little traffic; the main danger which a person here has to fear from others is an attack by soldiers or thieves. When people look around them, scanning the trees and hills or the road itself, they do so primarily because they must always be prepared for armed attack, and only secondarily because they have to avoid collision, on the main roads of this society demands a constant readiness to fight, and free play of the emotions in defence of one's life or possessions from physical attack.
>
> (Elias 1939: 368)

Increased interdependence between people, free competition, the monopolies of physical force and finance, growing social differentiation and the progressive division of functions led to the need for more stable and uniform behaviour. The psychic inscription of self-control mechanisms functioning automatically assisted in this regulatory process without the need for external coercion, making it the individual's own responsibility to act in a correct and acceptable way and prevent any movement that could be considered transgressive by society. Therefore, on a road like one of our time, we do not need to be constantly prepared to react against any kind of violent attack. These, when they happen and even though they may be frequent, are, most of the time unexpected and uncontrollable reactions and cannot be considered a normal pattern of behaviour. We circulate in public spaces far less unconcerned about attacks of violence than was the case in past centuries. Elias continues,

> Traffic on the main roads of a big city in the differentiated society of our time, by contrast, demands a quire different moulding of the psychological apparatus. Here the danger of physical arrack is minimal. Cars are rushing in all direction; pedestrians and cyclists are trying to thread their way through the *mêlée* of cars; policemen stand at the main crossroads to regulate the traffic with varying success.
>
> (Elias 1939: 368)

Throughout the civilizing process, people broaden the scope of identification with each other, consequently increasing the pressure for prestige and power. Relationships become ever closer, even those that need to cross oceans of distance, and more synchronized with the *rhythms* of a certain era. This rhythm, so often criticized as maddening, indicates the enormous number of interdependent relationships, which apply a constant competitive pressure on individuals. Individuals always have to anticipate and organize their actions in the long-term in order to avoid any kind of disturbance that might produce a threat to their social position.

In this long civilizing process, the distance between one class and another diminish and, therefore, so do the contrasts between their members. Habits and standards of conduct become increasingly similar among individuals of different social strata, just as the lower and upper classes slowly become similar to each other. This closeness creates a constant pressure between the upper and lower groups, through a game of competition for opportunities and for prestige that forces the higher group to establish marks of distinction:

> For the court nobility, too, the self-restraint imposed on them by their function and situation served at the same time as a prestige value, a means of distinguishing themself from the lower groups harrying them, and they did everything within their power to prevent these differences from being effaced.
>
> (Elias 1939: 387)

Faced with the context of tension produced in the relationship between the different classes, individuals feel threatened of losing their special position, whether through the irruption of feelings and passions, or through transgressive behaviour.

Little by little, the customs of the upper classes are disseminated among the lower classes that, in their desire to rise in social status, assume the characteristics of the more privileged groups, incorporating their habits and reproducing their institutions. For example, in the analysis of the formation of court society, Elias verifies that the complexification of the networks of interdependence led to an interpenetration of the standards of conduct of the nobility and the bourgeoisie. The bourgeoisie put pressure on the nobility, seeking equal prestige and recognition. In the same way, a part of the nobility approached the king and became more dependent on him. In this way, they could have access to a nobler life, with more economic opportunities and more differentiation from the lower classes.

The closeness to the king and the distance from the bourgeoisie gave meaning to the life of the nobles so that the anxiety at the loss of a higher social status produced a *desire for social prestige* that, in the end, contributed to distinguishing themselves from the lower social classes. In this way, the contact, proximity, and functional integration between the nobility and the bourgeoisie established a game of tensions in which each party strove to seek a balance.

The reduction of the contrasts between social classes, as occurred in the transition from warriors to courtiers, when the urban bourgeoisie came to be much closer to the nobility and to create games of competition with it, began to produce a pressure from below that threatened the monopoly of the court government. At the same time as the standard of living of the lower classes increased, habits peculiar to the upper classes were also established, which served to form social distinctions. Customs, gestures, dress, and entertainment established a chasm over the social pressure that was produced by reducing the differences between classes.

> It was this very distance from the bourgeoisie, their character as nobles, their membership of the upper class of the country, that gave their lives meaning and direction. The desire to preserve their class prestige, to "distinguish" themselves, motivated their actions far more than the desire to accumulate money.
>
> (Elias 1939: 395)

What really interested the nobility were not the economic accumulations, which could be obtained by various means, but the condition of prestige that differentiated them from the other social strata, thus linking the economic factor with a certain standard of living. The self-discipline that appears in the form of control of emotions and behaviour served to characterize the life of the good society. Among the changes in the structure of human relations, transformations in the psychic economy of individuals were also involved.

This does not mean that there was no form of self-control in medieval warrior societies or in any other society that was not organized in a centralizing instance of power. The self-regulation of individuals who made up these societies is more diffuse, unstable and restricted to acts of physical violence and to more abrupt emotional manifestations. Even with the decrease in physical violence between human relations, life does not become completely peaceful. Violence, which used to come in the form of aggression and physical threats, turns into pressure and competition for prestige. "If the sword no longer plays so great a role as the means of decision, it is replaced by intrigue", says Elias, "conflicts in which careers and social success are contested with words" (Elias 1939: 398). The violence that once operated physically between individuals now operates within the psychic sphere of individuals.

The process that led to the formation of modern states corresponded to some changes in the personality structure and affective life of individuals or, to use a Freudian expression, in the destinies of drives. In the face of these considerations, violence enters vertically, inscribed as an intrinsic element in the process of civilization. The spontaneous manifestations of the drive are recalled, everything that is of the order of aggressiveness and sexuality is transferred to another sphere, far from public life and away from the eyes of all others. Thus, an external conflict starts to operate as a psychic conflict and the superego acts as the instance which regulates a part of the violence and sexuality, which previously was more freely discharged in the external world, behind the psychic scene.

The fourth and last part of *The Civilizing Process*, entitled "Synopsis: Toward a Theory of Civilizing Processes", is more than a synopsis or a recap of all the ideas presented throughout the work. At this point, Elias turns to Freudian theory in a more forceful way. With the appropriation of psychoanalytic concepts, he shows how the transformations in the social structures, especially in the passage from the feudal period to the formation of modern absolutist states, implied changes in the psychic economy of individuals – regarding the self-regulating mechanisms and the production of affections – which led to the formation of the structure of the psychic apparatus as proposed by Freud in the early 20th century.

The hypothesis that the building of civilization is done by the repression of drives brings Norbert Elias's thought closer to Sigmund Freud's theory. For the psychoanalyst, the interdictions that society exerts on individuals enable the establishment of social ties. In *Thoughts for the Times on War and Death* [*Zeitgemäßes über Krieg und Tod*], written in 1915, Freud analyzes, as a direct witness of the events, the changes that the horrors of World War I produced on our illusions and our attitude towards death. Until that moment, civilized states seemed to hold themselves up to the highest moral standards, being intolerant of any individual who dared to violate them. It was to be assumed, in this sense, that even states themselves were subordinate to the moral principles which supported their demands.

In this text, Freud recognizes that it is the function of the state to control violence and the economy with a view to more stable and peaceful social pacts between individuals. It would be up to civilized states to prohibit individuals from acting unjustly, "not because it desires to abolish it, but because it desires to monopolize it, like salt and tobacco" (Freud 1915: 279), says Freud, full of a certain complaint about the difficult access to his main vice. This does not mean that, in times of war, the state itself could not behave unjustly. Previous wars, on the contrary, served to indicate the progress of civilization. The violence produced in these times of unrest was not capable of breaking the ethical relations and moral standards established for itself and its citizens. But with the First War, the war they feared so much came and produced the greatest disillusionment in the progress of civilization. A bloody, destructive, cruel and ruthless war.

Even if wars momentarily suspended the actions of repression, for Freud, civilization has always been sustained by the guarantee of regulating drives, so that the *aptitude for culture*, as Freud characterizes the human being's tendency to direct himself towards others, is due to the action of two factors: the internal factor, by which the individual seeks love and recognition from other people in order to be able to live, modifying his egoistic investments into social investments; the external factor, which refers to the learning capacity, by which individuals are subjected to the forces of the coercions of the environment. In this perspective, "Throughout an individual's life there is a constant replacement of external by internal compulsion" (Freud 1915: 69). The joint action of these two elements leads to what we could call the *Freudian civilizing process*. And, in a hypothesis that is fundamental to Elias's thesis on the civilizing process, Freud states,

> In the last resort it may be assumed that every internal compulsion which makes itself felt in the development of human beings was originally – that is, in the *history of mankind* – only an external one. Those who are born to-day bring with them as an inherited organization some degree of tendency (disposition) towards the transformation of egotistic into social instincts, and this disposition is easily stimulated into bringing about that result. A further portion of this instinctual transformation has to be accomplished during the life of the individual himself. So the human being is subject not only to the pressure of his immediate cultural environment, but also to the influence of the cultural history of his ancestors.
>
> (Freud 1915: 69–70)

Society ends up demanding from individuals a moral obedience that distances them from their own natural impulses. On each one of them relapses a merciless repression of the drives, which invariably results in the production of symptoms. The main points that allow us to define the direction of the civilizing process, as Elias demonstrates in the last part of *The Civilizing Process*, concern a series of transformations: the change of balance of external coercions into self-coercions; the emergence of social patterns of behaviour, which produce more automatic and more complete mechanisms of self-control; the increase in identification between individuals; the oscillations of expressions of emotions, which become less accentuated and more predictable; the notion between what is permitted to do in public or private spaces; the increase in the threshold of shame and repugnance in the face of certain behaviours and emotions.

The civilizing process has a direction that follows the balance between external coercions and self-coercions, which implies the settling of individual mechanisms to control drives, which become less vulnerable and less dependent on society's controls. The more stable and autonomous the psychic instances of self-coercion are, the more advanced is the civilizing process and the more balanced becomes the integration between individuals. However, we must remember that the theory on the civilizing process will consider its movements of advances and retreats, of control and flexibilization, of integration and disintegration, of pacification and violence so that the slightest force that unbalances this balance makes decivilizing movements resurface leading to the state of what is usually considered barbarism.

Changes in social grammar produce new psychic economies. In the passage from warrior society to court society, one leaves behind a life full of freedom, in which one was more accustomed to pass from one extreme to the other in one's affections, but also of threats and physical violence, in which passions and hatreds were satisfied without many limits. In its place, a more stable, more controlled life emerges, less threatened by dangers, unforeseen events and insecurities. The stabilization of this system by the monopoly of violence by the state inscribes in individuals' mechanisms of psychic self-control as a *second nature*.

> The controlling agency forming itself as part of the individual's personality structure corresponds to the controlling agency forming itself in society at large. The one like the other rends to impose a highly differentiated regulation upon all passionate impulses, upon people's conduce all around. Both – each to a large extent mediated by the other – exert a constant, even pressure to inhibit affective outbursts. They damp down extreme fluctuations in behaviour and emotions.
>
> (Elias 1939: 373)

The state's monopoly on the legitimate use of physical force protected individuals from the threat they posed to others. Life became more stable and individuals ceased to be at the mercy of sudden changes in affections. However, the transfer of control of violence to the State did not imply its annulment in social ties, much less in the drive economy. Violence relating to the other, which before occurred without control or predictability, turned to the individual in the form of psychic conflicts and the production of symptoms. In Elias's words,

> But at the same time the battlefield is, in a sense, moved within. Part of the tensions and passions that were earlier directly released in the struggle of man and man, must now be worked out within the human being. The more peaceful constraints exerted on people by their relations to others are mirrored within; an individualized pattern of near-automatic habits is established and consolidated, a specific "super-ego", which endeavours to control, transform or suppress his or her affects in keeping with the social structure.
>
> (Elias 1939: 375)

And so, the control of violence, when internalized in individuals, became the responsibility of the superegoic instance, which, in turn, as a representative of social coercions, acts violently against unconscious desires and against the pulsional forces of the individual, bringing about a permanent interior restlessness. Elias continues,

> But the drives, the passionate affects, that can no longer directly manifest themselves in the relationships *between* people, often struggle no less violently *within* the individual against this supervising part of themselves. And this semi-automatic struggle of the person with him or herself does not

> always find a happy resolution; the self-transformation required by life in this society does not always lead to a new balance between drive-satisfaction and drive-control.
>
> (Elias 1939: 375)

Thus, in face of a new social grammar of the court, the discontent becomes an immanent condition of the relationship between "individual" and "society", inscribing a wall between these terms. The drive will never cease its source and its strength, in the same way that social relations can never satisfy the goals of the drives. Once again, Elias corroborates Freudian propositions:

> The vertical oscillations, if we may so describe them, the leaps from fear to joy, pleasure to remorse are reduced, while the horizontal fissure running right through the whole person, the tension between the "super-ego" and the "unconscious" or "subconscious" – the wishes and desires that cannot be remembered – increases.
>
> (Elias 1939: 375)

People lead their lives in constant restlessness, in so far as drives can only be satisfied in deviant destinations, such as in fantasies and dreams. The feeling of guilt also expresses that the desires of the individual can no longer be said for oneself, nor for others who live with him. With the fear of transgressing social norms, one fears losing the love and respect of the people to whom he attributes high value. Social anxieties indicate the fears of individuals of being excluded from privileged social ties. Standards of distinction between normality and abnormality socially constituted through what is expected and planned about what is or is not accepted become naturalized.

2.4 Superego controls and a new psychic economy of the court

Without any doubt, it was in Freud's second topic, especially regarding the elaboration of the concept of superego, where Norbert Elias found elements that enabled the development of his theory of the civilizing process. From the text *The Ego and the Id* [*Das Ich und das Es*], of 1923, Freud establishes a new typology for the instances of the psychic apparatus, no longer divided between unconscious, conscious, and preconscious, but now between ego, id, and superego. In chapter III, by analyzing states of mourning, Freud describes the formation of the superego by the process of differentiation of the ego, a modification that is produced by the identification of the ego with a love relationship that has been lost.

For Freud, it was not any lost that led to the formation of the superego, but the first and most significant identification of the individual: "with the father in his own personal prehistory" (Freud 1923: 31). The superego corresponds to this first model of identification of the child with its father: "When the ego assumes the features of the object, it is forcing itself, so to speak, upon the id as a love-object and is trying to make good the id's loss by saying: 'Look, you can love me too – I am so like the object'" (Freud 1923: 30). It does not fall to the superego, however, only the function of imposing ways of being: "You *ought to be* like this (like your father)", but also of placing certain prohibitions: "You *may not be* like this (like your father) – that is, you may not do all that he does; some things are his prerogative" (Freud 1923: 34).

To the superego, the psychic instance that represents the paternal insignia corresponds two functions. First, it acts as the origin of ethical, aesthetic and social commandments, which determine values, rules, and tastes to be followed. Secondly, it serves as a coercive instance, which establishes impediments to the realization of, particularly those that Freud calls oedipal, insofar as they inscribe the individual in social ties.

> The ego ideal is therefore the heir of the Oedipus complex, and thus it is also the expression of the most powerful impulses and most important libidinal vicissitudes of the id. By setting up this ego ideal, the ego has mastered the Oedipus complex and at the same time placed itself in subjection to the id. Whereas the ego is essentially the representative of the external world, of reality, the super-ego stands in contrast to it as the representative of the internal world, of the id. Conflicts between the ego and the ideal will, as we are now prepared to find, ultimately reflect the contrast between what is real and what is psychical, between the external world and the internal world.
>
> (Freud 1923: 38)

The superego is not in a position of dependence with the external world, as one might imagine due to its function of representing the highest civilizing values of humanity. By placing itself as an ideal model which attracts the main libidinal investments of the ego, it places itself at the service of the impulses. The superego, in the dimension which situates it as an ego ideal, represents everything that the ego aspires to be. The ego is formed, then, by the abandoned investments of the id – which first and foremost came to constitute the superego. It is in this sense that Freud affirms that the superego knows more about the unconscious than the ego itself. The ego seeks to control the investments of the id by means of the superego. The energy that reaches the superego comes directly from the impulses, so that it is charged by both sexual impulses and aggressive impulses. From the superego, we see falling on the ego a parcel of love and death.

> But the derivation of the super-ego from the first object-cathexes of the id, from the Oedipus complex, signifies even more for it. This derivation, as we have already shown, brings it into relation with the phylogenetic acquisitions of the id and makes it a reincarnation of former egostructures which have left their precipitates behind in the id. Thus the super-ego is always close to the id and can act as its representative *vis-à-vis* the ego. It reaches deep down into the id and for that reason is farther from consciousness than the ego is.
>
> (Freud 1923: 48)

Because it is subjugated to the actions of the superego, the ego fears being hated and abandoned by it, being left at the mercy of death itself. The fear of death, then, no longer takes place between the ego and the external world, but between the ego and the superego. At the same time: "To the ego, therefore, living means the same as being loved by the super-ego, which here again appears as the representative of the id" (Freud 1923: 58). The superego, in this sense, performs the same function as the father of a small child, divine providence or fate, namely that of protecting and giving love.

The problem of the transmission of the cultural inheritance, then, poses itself as a question for Freud. Would the inherited content pass from individual to individual in a hereditary way through the ego or through the id? At once, Freud answers that the unconscious would be incapable of recording experiences except through the actions of the ego. However, one cannot speak of a hereditary transmission in the ego, insofar as it is a part of the id that has differentiated itself. Freud remains with the interrogation, but launches the basis for some hypotheses that, in less than ten years, helped Norbert Elias to elaborate his theory on the process of transmission of social rules and norms by the formation and sharing of habits. Freud, then, launches his ideas:

> The experiences of the ego seem at first to be lost for inheritance; but, when they have been repeated often enough and with sufficient strength in many individuals in successive generations, they transform themselves, so to say, into experiences of the id, the impressions of which are preserved by heredity. Thus in the id, which is capable of being inherited, are harboured residues of the existences of countless egos; and, when the ego forms its super-ego out of the id, it may perhaps only be reviving shapes of former egos and be bringing them to resurrection.
>
> (Freud 1923: 38)

The experiences of the ego, when repeated with sufficient *frequency* and *force*, says Freud, are inscribed in the unconscious as part of it. Certain habits that were first instituted as external social rules, dictating ways of feeling and behaving, become inscribed in the unconscious and are transmitted over generations without the subject knowing it. If the superego is a representative of the id and the drives, as Freud observed, it is possible to say that patterns of the unconscious are transmitted by the superego itself, in such a way that our highest civilizing values are intimately linked to the most archaic of drives. This is why the superego plays a fundamental role in the psychic constitution and in the formation of social institutions. On the one hand, the entrance in the social ties is linked to unconscious narcissistic conditions. On the other hand, social ties provide the identification traces in which the subject finds or does not find his or her place of belonging.

In the 31st of the *New Introductory Lectures on Psychoanalysis* [*Neue Folge der Vorlesungen zur Einführung in die Psychoanalyse*], in 1933, about the split of the psychic personality, Freud resumes the ego as a psychic instance whose boundaries with the internal and external worlds are not rigidly established. Like a crystal thrown to the ground, which shatters according to the lines of separation, the ego is also organized as a structure marked by cracks and ruptures which end up articulating themselves as elements of connection between one and the other. This is what happens with the superego, a psychic instance differentiated from the ego which, in certain structures or situations, such as paranoia and jealousy, is transferred to the external world as if it were not part of the individual.

What stands out from the elements added by Freud to the theory on the superego is the process of transmission of culture. It is the function of the superego to pass on, between generations, the elements of civilization, insofar as the superego results from the identification of the ego with another individual as a model not through his ego, but through his superego:

> Thus a child's super-ego is in fact constructed on the model not of its parents but of its parents' super-ego; the contents which fill it are the same and it becomes the vehicle of tradition and of all the time-resisting judgements of values which have propagated themselves from generation to generation.
> (Freud 1933: 67)

In this way, Freud addresses an important problem concerning the question of the unconscious transmission of cultural elements, without having to resort to the hypothesis of hereditary transmission.

To what Norbert Elias explains by means of the formation of habits, in the form of a *second nature* or an *embodied social knowledge*, which are taught and transmitted unconsciously between people of different generations, Freud replies that it is up to the superego to understand human social conduct. Freud's fundamental addition to the theory of the superego is that the boundaries and distinctions of the psychic instances are also not well established, so that "As you see here, the super-ego merges into the id; indeed, as heir of the Oedipus complex it has intimate relations with the id" (Freud 1933: 79). Part of the superego, in this sense, operates unconsciously in the individual.

From the actions of the superego over the ego, Freud highlights the formation of two important unconscious feelings: the *sense of guilt* and the *feeling of inferiority*. If, for Freud, both are affections produced by the dynamics of the relations between the psychic instances, for Elias, moreover, they are results of a civilizing process whose transformation of social structures has engendered changes in the psychic economy of individuals. Both the guilt and the inferiority result from the tension between the ego and the superego.

Human beings become more complex to the extent that an internal conflict is established with oneself. The renunciation of the satisfaction of drives, the disguising of passions and the deviation of actions are essential changes for the maintenance of a certain social position, as Elias describes: "The 'world picture' gradually becomes less directly determined by human wishes and fears, and more strongly orientated to what we call 'experience' or 'the empirical', to sequences with their own immanent regularities" (Elias 1939: 400). As a result, there is a distancing between the ego and the other, who comes to be seen as an isolated individual who observes at the same time as he can also be observed, who controls at the same time as he is controlled, who dominates at the same time as he is dominated. It is in the court circle, according to Elias, that a "psychological human self-image developed", in which one seeks a "more precise observation of others and oneself in terms of longer series of motives and causal connections" (Elias 1939: 400). In this sense, one of the research proposals of *The Civilizing Process* is precisely to criticize the neutrality of the modern sciences, especially in relation to the sciences that came to develop in their experimental and laboratory branches.

It is a critique of the scientificity of psychology, history, and sociology in proposing themselves as sciences that seek to think of the human being as an isolated structure, independent of each other and possible to be studied separately. The possibility of observing and examining people and oneself places the individual under the condition of an absolute autonomy, with easily predictable behaviours and identifiable causes, without considering any effect of the social context. Thus, even appropriating psychoanalytical concepts for the development of his ideas, Norbert Elias already pointed out one of his main criticisms to Freud. For him, Freudian metapsychology also results from modern science by proposing the atemporality and a-historicity of the unconscious. Psychoanalysis, in Elias's reading, supports the possibility of determining a beginning for the emergence of civilization, an origin of individuals, thereby disregarding the social processes involved in the formation of psychic structures. Freudian theory, then, would have formulated a starting point for the individual, as well as for civilization. As we see in this passage from Elias,

> Our habits of thinking incline us to look for "beginnings'"; but there is in the development of human beings a "point" before which one could say that hitherto there was no *ratio* and now it has "*arisen*"; that hitherto there were no self-constraints and no "super-ego" and now, in this or that century, they are suddenly there. There is no zero-point to any of these data. But it does no more justice to the facts to say: everything was always there as it is now. The habits of self-constraint, the organization of consciousness and affects of "civilized" people, clearly differ *in their totality* from those of so-called "primitives"; but both are, in their structure, different yet clearly explainable mouldings of largely the same natural functions.
>
> (Elias 1939: 403)

The unconscious, the drives and the self-control mechanisms are productions that are socially organized. The difference in the psychic structure of individuals living in other times and other societies refers to the form and degree to which these elements are articulated, especially because the historical transformations increase the relations of dependence and the division of functions between individuals. In this sense, for Elias, it is possible to state that not only the *self-image*, but also a whole way of functioning of the drive economy distinguishes different social configurations by having gone through different processes of social and historical formation.

A second critical perspective of Elias to Freudian psychoanalysis concerns the idea that the different strata of the functioning of the mind could be studied separately. It would then be possible, for example, to isolate conscious thought and ideas from drives and affections. Modern psychoanalytic research, says Elias, "tends, in considering human beings, to extract something 'unconscious', conceived as an 'id' without history, as the most important element in the whole psychological structure" (Elias 1939: 409). While psychoanalytic clinical practice, according to him, seems to have more or less corrected itself to this conception, theory, continues the sociologist, still considers that

> the steering of the individual by unconscious libidinal impulses has a form and structure of its own, independently of the figurational destiny of the individual, the changing fortunes of his relationships with others throughout his life, and independently too of the pattern and structure of the other self-steering functions of his personality, conscious and unconscious. No distinction is made between the natural raw material of drives, which indeed perhaps changes little throughout the whole history of humankind, and the increasingly more firmly wrought structures of control, and thus the paths into which the elementary energies are channelled in each person through his or her relations with other people from birth onward.
>
> (Elias 1939: 403)

Elias seems to make an effort to introduce the drives not only into the functioning of the processes of thought, originating in the ego and the superego, but also into the historical-social processes that underlie the psychic constitution of the individual. Elias continues,

> The libidinal energies which one encounters in any living human being are always already socially processed; they are, in other words, sociogenetically transformed in their function and structure, and can in no way be separated from the corresponding ego and super-ego structures.
>
> (Elias 1939: 403)

It is as if the psychic structures, for Freud, did not suffer the influences of the various relationships that individuals constitute throughout their lives, nor of the learning processes, nor of the transformations in society. The unconscious, the drives and the defence mechanisms are all, in Elias's view, structures determined by history and social processes. Thus, what the sociologist calls animal and automatic levels of the human personality, in order to refer to the unconscious contents and drives, must be combined with the elements of social learning, responsible for the control of behaviours and affections.

Elias, then, takes up the idea that Freud had developed, in *Group Psychology and the Analysis of the Ego*, of 1921, and in *Inhibition, Symptom and Anxiety*, of 1926, about the function of the affections as a form of regulation of behaviours in order to maintain a forecast against the infraction of the codes of conduct so as not to threaten the position of the individual and the social class to which he belongs. The economy of affect cannot be separated from the process of formation of social structures. This hypothesis reinforces the idea that the drive, in its functioning as an on and off energy, is intimately inserted within social institutions.

> The fear arising from the situation of the whole group, from their struggle to preserve their cherished and threatened position, acts directly as a force maintaining the code of conduct, the cultivation of the super-ego in its members. It is converted into individual anxiety, the individual's fear of personal degradation or merely loss of prestige in his own society. And it is this fear of loss of prestige in the eyes of others, instilled as self-compulsion, whether in the form of shame or a sense of honour, which assures the habitual reproduction of distinctive conduct, and the strict drive-control underlying it, in individual people.
>
> (Elias 1939: 385)

Thus, in the last session of his general theory of the civilizing process, Elias investigates the circuit of affections in the civilizing process. Shame, guilt, fear, and repugnance are feelings that participate in the balance of power between the different parts that constitute societies. With the consolidation of court societies, it was possible to perceive an increase in the level of shame and repugnance, affections that are produced automatically from the establishment of certain habits and customs. Their function is not related, as we might think, to hygienist issues that would serve the preservation of the health of individuals, but rather they concern the condition of power, of belonging, and of occupation of places of privilege in a given social class, marking the limits of distinction and equality between those who are inside and those who are outside, those who belong and those who are excluded.

Affections are not individual productions, nor can they be reduced to the sphere of family relations, but are imbricated in the dynamics of the power games of social relations. In this sense, what is at issue in the production of shame and disgust is a fear of social degradation in the face of other people's superiority. Individual and society are mixed in the affections generated by social conflicts that are reproduced and transmitted in the form of psychic conflicts.

> The conflict expressed in shame-fear is nor merely a conflict of the individual with prevalent social opinion; the individual's behaviour has brought him into conflict with the part of himself that represents this social opinion. It is a conflict within his own personality; he himself recognizes himself as inferior. He fears the loss of the love or respect of others, to which he attaches or has attached value. Their attitude has precipitated an attitude within him that he automatically adopts towards himself. This is what makes him so defenceless against gestures of superiority by others which somehow trigger off this automatism within him.
>
> (Elias 1939: 415)

The superego results from a civilizing process that psychically installed in individuals a social conflict that naturalized a certain group or social class as superior, more powerful and with more privileges, in relation to a group or social class that was humanly inferior, originally submissive, and deservedly underprivileged. A power game of foreign policy that reproduces itself as a power game of domestic policy. In this sense, it is clear the effects of the increased division of social functions in the differentiation between psychic functions, drive, and mechanisms of drive control. The drives force, motivated by the search for satisfaction of unconscious desires, lead individuals to seek the rupture of social rules and of self-coercion imposed by themselves. We continue with Elias,

> The layer of psychological functions which, in the course of the social transformation that has been described, is gradually differentiated from the drives, the ego or superego functions, has, in other words, a twofold task within the personality: *they conduct at the same time a domestic policy and a foreign policy* – which, moreover, are not always in harmony and quite often are contradictory.
>
> (Elias 1939: 416 – emphasis in original)

Freud and Elias, in this view, seem to agree with each other. The advancement in this perspective, in 1908, the psychoanalyst even stated,

> But, far from this being so, I must insist upon that view that neuroses, whatever their extent and wherever they occur, always succeeds in frustrating the purpose of civilization, and in that way actually perform the work of the suppressed mental forces that are hostile to civilization.
>
> (Freud 1908: 202–203)

Paradoxically, the drive forces of individuals, which impel them towards the other in search of satisfaction of their desires, also produce resistance to social ties.

Notes

1 I evoke here the letter Sigmund Freud wrote to Wilhelm Fliess on 6 December 1896, known as *Letter 52*, where the psychoanalyst states, "As you know, I am working on the assumption that our psychic mechanism has come into being by a process of stratification: the material present in the form of memory traces being subjected from time to time to a rearrangement in accordance with fresh circumstances – to a *retranscription*. Thus, what is essentially new about my theory is the thesis that memory is present not once but several times over, that it is laid down in various kinds of indications" (Freud 1986: 207).

2 The relationship of individuals to death throughout the civilizing process was further explored and elaborated upon by Norbert Elias in his text *The Loneliness of the Dying*. Regarding the difference in attitude towards death, especially about the safety and predictability of death, between feudal and modern societies, Elias states, "In the more developed nation-states people's security, their protection against the more brutal strokes of fate such as illness and sudden death, is much greater than in earlier periods, and perhaps greater than at any time in the development of humanity. As compared with earlier stages, life

in these societies has become more predictable, while demanding from each individual a higher degree of foresight and control of the passions. The relatively high life expectancy of individuals in these societies is a reflection of the increased security. Among the knights of the thirteenth century a man of forty was counted almost an old man; in the industrial societies of the twentieth century he is considered almost young – with class specific differences. The prevention and treatment of illness in the present century are better organized than ever before, inadequate as they may still be. The internal pacification of society, the individual's protection against violence not sanctioned by the state, as against starvation, has reached a pitch unimaginable to people of earlier times" (Elias 1982: 07).

References

Benveniste, Émile (1966) *Problems in General Linguistics*. Miami: University of Miami Press, 1971.

De Quincey, Thomas (1827) "The Last Days of Immanuel Kant", in *The Last Days of Immanuel Kant and Other Writing*. Miami: HardPress, 2017.

Elias, Norbert (1938) "Elias to Benjamin", in D. Schöttker "Norbert Elias and Walter Benjamin: An Exchange of Letters and its Context", in *History of the Human Sciences*, vol. 11, n.2, pp. 45–59.

——— (1939) *The Civilizing Process. Sociogenetic and Psychogenetic Investigations*, ed. by E. Dunning, J. Goudsblom and S. Mennell, trans. by E. Japhcott. Oxford: Blackwell Publishing, 2013.

——— (1982) *The Loneliness of the Dying*, trans. by E. Jephcott. New York/London: Continuum, 2001.

——— (1987) *Norbert Elias: Reflections on a Life*. Cambridge: Polity Press, 1994.

Freud, Sigmund (1908) "'Civilized' Sexual Morality and Modern Nervous Illness", in *The Standard Edition of the Complete Psychological Works of Sigmund Freud – Jensen's 'Gradiva' and Other Works (1906–1908)*, vol. IX, ed. and trans. by J. Strachey. London: Hogarth Press, 1981.

——— (1915) "Thought for the Times on War and Death", in *The Standard Edition of the Complete Psychological Works of Sigmund Freud – On the History of Psycho-analytic Movement, Papers on Metapsychology and Other Works (1914–1916)*, vol. XIV, ed. and trans. by J. Strachey. London: Hogarth Press, 1981.

——— (1923) "The Ego and the Id", in *The Standard Edition of the Complete Psychological Works of Sigmund Freud – The Ego and the Id and Other Works (1923–1925)*, vol. XIX, ed. and trans. by J. Strachey. London: Hogarth Press, 1986.

——— (1933) "The Dissection of the Psychical Personality", in *The Standard Edition of the Complete Psychological Works of Sigmund Freud – New Introductory Lectures on Psychoanalysis and Other Works (1932–1936)*, vol. XXII, ed. and trans. by J. Strachey. London: Hogarth Press, 1981.

——— (1986) "Letter 52", in *The Complete Letters of Sigmund Freud to Wilhelm Fliess: 1887–1904*, ed. and trans. by J. M. Masson. London: Harvard University Press.

Rousseau, Jean-Jacques (1762) *The Social Contract*, trans. by M. Cranston. London: Penguins Book, 1968.

Weber, Max (1919) "Politics as a Vocation", in *The Vocations Lectures*, ed. by D. Owen and T. Strong, trans. by R. Livingstone. Cambridge: Hackett Publishing Company, 2004.

3 Logic of exclusion

The established and the outsiders

Throughout his life, wherever he went, Norbert Elias never ceased to be an outsider. Similarly, his work was never curtailed by any borders. Transiting through disciplines like sociology, history, psychoanalysis, philosophy, education, politics, the arts and sport, his research for many years and even today does not appear to have had a suitably wide reach. "Do we really understand Norbert Elias?" (Lacroix 1997: 31), Bernard Lacroix asks. By the end of his life the answer always seemed evident to Elias himself: "Actually, I still do not have the feeling that I am fully understood" (Elias 1987b: 73). In light of this, the dream that he claimed to recurrently have is of considerable significance:

> I am speaking into a telephone and the voice at the other end says, "Could you speak louder, I can't hear you", and then I start to shout, and the other voice keeps saying, "Speak louder, I can't hear you".
>
> (Elias 1987b: 72–73)

In the initial period of his exile in England, Elias was awarded a research grant at the London School of Economics, transferred to Cambridge after the outbreak of World War II and financed by the Rockefeller Foundation until June 1944. It was only in 1954 that he managed to secure his first university teaching position. Before that, Elias survived outside the university realm, despite his previous experience in Germany. In London he was part of a very intense circle of German intellectuals of Jewish origin. For many years he was invited to the Christmas celebrations hosted by Francis Ludwig Carsten, a British historian with an interest in Nazi Germany, also attended by George Mosse, an American historian of German origin, who came to be a leading reference on the concept of the brutalisation of European societies in the inter-war period. Gisèle Freund, an important photographer and sociologist, whom Elias had met in Frankfurt, where he had recommended her to write what came to be her work *French Photography in the 19th Century*, was also a member of this circle of friends during the early years of her exile in England.

In this context of friendship ties, a 20-page article was published in 1950 in the *British Journal of Sociology* entitled *Studies in the Genesis of the Naval Profession* (Elias 1950). This would prove to be the first essay on how Elias's relational sociology covers the formation process of the British State via the sociogenesis of

DOI: 10.4324/9781003378938-3

the naval profession. Elias linked the training for this new profession to the state's demand to hold a monopoly of violence in the naval realm, sustained by rivalry between two divergent groups – professional seamen gentlemen officers – in a power struggle between two previously independent professions.

Norbert Elias also participated in group analysis activities organized by the psychoanalyst Siegmund Heinrich Foulkes. A German psychiatrist of Jewish origin, Foulkes who was born with the surname Fuchs, studied medicine at the universities of Heidelberg and Frankfurt. In 1928 he went to Vienna to begin his training in psychoanalysis at the Vienna Psychoanalytic Society. Since the sale and export of tobacco were regulated by the Austrian government and the only cigars available in Viennese tobacconists [*Trafiks*] were a state monopoly, the occasional cigar smoked by Freud ended up being smuggled by Foulkes via his friend Karl Landauer, one of the founders of the *Frankfurt School*.

As Foulkes recounts in the text *Recollections of my visit to Freud* (Foulkes 1969), he only managed to meet Sigmund Freud in person in 1936, at the summer residence of the Freud family in Grinzing, a small community about 20 kilometres from Vienna, later subsumed within the capital city. On the eve of his 80th birthday, Freud still wished to remain in Vienna: "No, we will stay here. We have accommodated ourselves as if nothing was amiss" (Freud *quoted* Foulkes 1969: 25), was supposedly his response to Foulkes when asked if he felt safe in Austria. Freud appeared to be an optimistic sceptic, still confident about a future that soon proved to be a dark one: "We shall get by; it is not likely that things here will be as brutal as in Germany" (Freud *quoted* Foulkes 1969: 25), he told Foulkes.

Analyzed by Hélène Deutsch in Vienna, Foulkes attended Wilhelm Reich's seminars and in the 1930s joined the recently formed Frankfurt Psychoanalytic Institute. In 1933, with the rise of the Nazi party, he sought refuge in England at the invitation of Ernest Jones, soon joining the British Psychoanalytical Society. Foulkes, who already knew Elias from the time the two of them lived in Frankfurt, was one of the first psychoanalysts to read the work *The Civilizing Process*, even writing a review of the book that was published in German and English. Despite some criticisms of the work's psychological dimension, he was interested in writing a book with Elias about the relationships between psychoanalysis and sociology.

In 1948 Foulkes had brought together a group of psychiatrists and psychotherapists to hold an international congress about mental illness that included professionals from other disciplines, like sociology and anthropology. He therefore approached Elias to form part of his interdisciplinary group and thus be able to establish the theoretical bases of group analysis. After the congress the group continued to meet. Elias was the only sociologist in a group of psychoanalysts, in a permanent tension in his relationship with the group.

In Foulkes's opinion, in group analysis we do not observe the same processes that stem from the repetition of a child's Oedipus complex witnessed in individual analysis. He also called other phenomena into question. In his article "On group analysis", of 1946, he states that the free association method, the only rule put forward by Freud for practitioners of psychoanalysis, is only useful in group analysis in specific circumstances. The phenomenon of transference, resistance, and other defence mechanisms are also part of group analysis. Everything else is different, in his view. Foulkes endeavoured to clearly establish the divisions between the two forms of treatment, in order to keep Freudian technique and theory intact and to necessitate the creation of concepts for group experiences. In *The group as a matrix of the individual's mental life*, of 1971, Foulkes seems to distance himself from Freudian conceptualisations by suggesting that the psychoanalytical perspective considers an individual's mind as a unit whose processes are understood in individual terms. In Foulkes's words,

> As group analysts we do not share the psychoanalytical juxtaposition of an "internal" psychological reality and an "external", physical or social reality which, for psychoanalysis, makes good sense. What is inside is outside, the "social" is not external but very much internal too and penetrates the innermost being of the individual personality. The "objective" external "reality" is inseparable from the being, animal or human, and indeed the individual whose world it is and therefore is part of the "psychological" reality as well.
> (Foulkes 1971: 226–227)

Foulkes continues to put forward criticisms of psychoanalysis that resemble the critiques that Norbert Elias himself directed at Freudian theory. Psychoanalysis, for Foulkes, treats the individual deliberately as an abstraction, isolated from their context. He contends that, from a psychoanalytical point of view, the individual is often considered as an absolute truth, in which the patient's account is a truth that relates to just the mind of one individual. In this way, experiences of group analysis led him to believe in the existence of a suprapersonal and transpersonal *mental matrix*. The function of the concept of a matrix used by Foulkes – that often serves to describe the group's verbal and non-verbal context, the background that the individual is part of, a field of mental events that involve and go beyond the individual – harks back to Norbert Elias's concept of configurations, in that both aim to break with the notion of the individual as an entity isolated from other individuals. What is established are not relationships between independent beings, but mental processes that interact unconsciously in accordance with people's predisposition to determine their interactions.

In this context, in 1954 Elias received two offers of academic work. One in Leeds the other in Leicester. He chose Leicester due to its proximity to London and the British Museum. In the sociology department, the sociologists who went to teach there after Elias's arrival included Anthony Giddens and Eric Dunning. The latter, a young man encouraged by Elias to continue his studies about sport and violence, became one of the most important sociologists on the relationship between sport and the civilizing process and with Elias he published a series of studies on the sociology of sport applying the theory of civilizing processes.

3.1 Integrate and exclude

During the almost 40 years that he lived in England, one of Norbert Elias's most important works was the book *The Established and the Outsiders: A Sociological Enquiry into Community Problems*, in partnership with Professor John L. Scotson, his supervisor at the University of Leicester. The research that gave rise to this study was carried out in the late 1950s and early 1960s, in a small English community given the fictional name of Winston Parva. It was published for the first time in 1965, when Elias was still working as a teacher. If the authors' initial objective was to investigate teenage delinquency in this small place, the study ended up progressively focusing on the processes of social exclusion and stigmatization, the relationships of violence and power among its inhabitants – who differentiated themselves, as the authors termed them, as 'established' groups and 'outsider' groups.

The book *The Established and the Outsiders* can only be understood as the development of formulations about the civilizing process, seen as part of the collection of principal texts that make up Elias's intellectual production. Therefore, as Stephen Mennell writes,

> Both [the theory of established-outsiders relations and theory of the civilizing process] are concerned with the connections between the development of power relations and developments in personality structure, and both have proved valuable in a wide range of sociological investigations.
>
> (Mennell 1989: 137)

The theme of social exclusion was always a constant in Elias's work. *The Court Society*, written in the 1930s, is a good example of this. In this book Elias already outlined the logic of distinction in the formation of the French absolutist state, which pitched the former court aristocracy in competition with a new bourgeois class.

> Seen from the standpoint of court society the people of the professional strata are outsiders. They exist in the margin of the *monde* – the word is revealing – in the margin of the "great world". They are little people. Their houses lack the public, ostentatious character of the *hôtels* and palaces. They are private houses without significance, like their occupants.
>
> (Elias 1969: 55)

In this particular historical context, it was the new social class, the bourgeoisie, who were excluded by the members of court society, who had held power and the economic monopoly for centuries. To be able to distinguish itself socially, the French court created symbolic distances, creating its own manuals of etiquette and good conduct, marking on their bodies, affects, and gestures the value codifications that discriminated against and stigmatized those who did not obey the same rules. Even the king was obliged to comply with the excesses of these rituals, as we can see in the descriptions of Louis XIV's daily ceremonies of *lever* and *coucher*.

Court society created a courtly way of being that included a *habitus* solely for this class, constraining spontaneity in behaviour and emotions. The notion of *habitus* used by Elias corresponds to the psychological internalization of social norms and rules for the purpose of self-regulation, designating what he called "second nature" or an incorporated social knowledge. Consequently, every individual reproduces and passes on values in accordance with the social norms of the groups they are subjected to.

Through studying court society, Elias discovered the dual purpose of the formation of habitus: to *integrate* its members and to *exclude* others who did not incorporate the same ways of being. In the case of court society, exclusion served to signal social distinctions, public recognition and prestige. Social power enabled the establishment of its own codes and rules of conduct, through which different values were attributed to the existence of individuals depending on whether they were subjected to them or not. In this logic of distinction, the doors upward would always be open whereas the doors downward would always be closed.

At the root of these ideas is the repression of urges, transferring to the background of consciousness and private life all that does not fit the hegemonic structures of rationality and power. Linking social processes and the psychic economy of individuals, the configuration between established groups and outsiders supports a reality of social exclusion based on unconscious collective fantasies, since, as we will later see, social values impact on the influence that the *we-image* and the *we-ideal* have on the *self-image* and the *self-ideal*.

The research that Elias and Scotson carried out in Winston Parva illustrated not only the exclusion process between established groups and outsiders, but also revealed a universal theme about human relationships. Between social classes, races, religions, genders or nationalities, there will always be conflicts between groups of people who see themselves as superior being, blessed with better qualities, and groups of people considered inferior, lacking in virtues and less human. In light of this, the authors proposed to answer the following question:

> How is it done? How do members of a group maintain among themselves the belief that they are not merely more powerful but also better human beings than those of another? What means do they use to impose the belief in their own human superiority upon those who are less powerful?
>
> (Elias and Scotson 1965: xvi)

To explore these questions, the terms "established" and "outsiders" confer a relational specificity between the groups in this small English community. By using these terms, the authors distanced the explanation of social exclusions from Marxist and Weberian approaches, which predominated in 20th-century sociology, refusing to reduce these relationships to economic power, social class or any typology of domination. The recognition, by Elias himself, of the importance of Freud's thinking on his theory on the civilizing process makes it legitimate to assume the influence of psychoanalysis also on his research about the established/outsiders' configuration. However, in relation to the influence of Freudian thought on Elias's work, Mennell also states the following: "Elias uses Freudian vocabular – ego and super-ego, drives, libido, unconscious, repression and so on – in discussing psychological changes in the course of the civilizing process. This vocabular is more prominent in this early work than later" (Mennell 1989: 100). We can see the effects that psychoanalysis had not only on his research on the established/outsiders relational model, but also throughout his works from later periods of his life, advancing our understanding of the relationship between the individual and collective processes. We should not forget that the last text that Elias wrote before his death was precisely an open dialogue on the Freudian conception of society.

Stephen Mennell appears to agree with Elias's view of psychoanalysis, which reduces Freudian theory to the individual perspective and to the private life of the family sphere, and even naturalizes psychic processes that are constructed in the relationship that individuals establish with societies. Thus, referring to the reach of Elias's work, Mennell continues: "Collective fantasies have to be understood in the context of fluctuating power relations and tensions in figurations encompassing families of origin but going way beyond them in complexity and scope" (Mennell 1989: 139). Nevertheless, if the private structure of the family presents itself as one of the foundations of the psychic constitution, we cannot say that Freud did not consider the relationships of individuals with major social institutions, like the army and the church, which are analyzed in particular in his text *Group Psychology and the Analysis of the Ego*, of 1921.

The Winston Parva study deals above all with the human condition that, determined by the different configurations that people establish among themselves, cannot be considered an essence in itself. This small community, established in the 1880s by a businessman who built houses, factories and commercial outlets, was divided into three distinct zones:

- *Zone 2*, the oldest neighbourhood, known as the *village*, which was occupied by the first families who came to work in the region. Strong bonds of solidarity united the inhabitants of this zone, since its long-standing nature created an affective intimacy between them via long-lasting friendships and the sharing of common experiences.
- *Zone 1* corresponded to a residential neighbourhood that was built between the 1920s and 1930s. It was considered the most prestigious area and, with the passage of time, the inhabitants of Zone 2 who prospered and accumulated money moved here, with the result that some members of a single family lived in both these areas.
- *Zone 3*, in turn, had been built in the 1930s by other businessmen, in a swampy area full of rats; for this reason, the villagers called it *rat alley*. Due to military strategies during World War II, this third zone ended up receiving a wave of immigration made up of people made homeless by aerial bombings or people who were coming to work in the new factories.

The research carried out in Winston Parva showed that there were no differences of nationality, religion, ethnicity, colour, or race between the inhabitants of the three areas. Neither did they differentiate themselves from each other by profession, with their income, social class and educational level being very similar. In addition, there were no significant differences between the quality of their housing. However, Elias and Scotson found that the residents of one of the zones judged themselves to be superior to those from another zone. They saw themselves as better people, as members of a group with more charisma and power. They therefore refused to maintain contact with members of the other areas, whom they considered inferior as human beings. The main difference detected between the groups was the length of time they had lived there: the fact that some had arrived earlier than others. The residents of the area made up of the oldest families considered themselves superior human beings to the residents of the other areas, who were even treated as individuals from an inferior species. They did not allow anyone new to join their group, excluding all the other neighbours from non-professional social contact. Thus, a taboo was created with regard to the outsiders by creating gossip and stigmatizations.

The temporal factor was enough for a group to form more cohesive, more consolidated relationships with a greater degree of identification among their members. The places that each individual could occupy were determined by tradition. The shared lifestyle and the set of common norms and patterns of behaviour gave a sense of pride to the established members, and consequently the ties between the families became more stable and cohesive. To preserve the satisfaction and honour of belonging to a group of such high value, they created social barriers to keep anyone else out. The established reserved for themselves, their family members and friends the most privileged public positions, denying access to all those who were not part of the same social circle. This kind of corruption, in which the individual takes on state level positions through family ties, close friendships, or class similarities, is the residue of an ethos of societies that reduce the plurality of the collective to their identity.

To preserve one's own identity and have social control, the established attributed to themselves the sense of being immensely superior and stigmatized the outsiders via degrading labels. The individuals from the zones they looked down on in turn accepted resignedly this position of scorn, representing themselves as people of less value, bad, dirty, poor and dishonourable. In this sense "The complementarity of group charisma (one's own) and group disgrace (that of others) is one of the most significant aspects of the type of established-outsider relationship that one encounters here" (Elias and Scotson 1965: xxii). What we are dealing with here is a power relation with a *double link*, in which one side can only exist with the counterpoint of the other. The act of looking down on others is essential not only to sustain the position of privilege, but also as a way of finding purposes for what is unbearable about oneself.

How then can the need of the established to stigmatize the outsiders as people of less value be justified? What advantages encourage them to maintain their superior image at any cost? The transformation of something strange into a taboo is a topic that relates to Freud's research. In 1913, Freud dedicated his work *Totem and Taboo: Some Points of Agreement between the Mental Lives of Savages and Neurotics* [*Totem und tabu – Einige Übereinstimmungen im Seelenleben der Wilden und der Neurotiker*] to dealing with taboos as organizing elements of the social and psychic life of individuals. Regarding its origin, the word taboo simultaneously referred to a common trait shared by two different things, the *sacred* and the *impure*, reflecting the ambivalence of this dual meaning. Back in 1910, in the text *The Antithetical Meaning of Primal Words* [*Über den Gegensinn der Unworte*], Freud showed that in some ancient languages there were words that expressed two opposing meanings simultaneously, like strong and weak, good and bad, illuminated and dark. *Sacer*, for example, is a word that referred both to what is "holy, consecrated", and to what is "disturbing, strange, dangerous, impure". Subsequently, these antithetical meanings were separated, coming to refer to different objects.

According to *Totem and Taboo*, taboos are the product of affective ambivalence. They project unconscious hostility onto an adored object, transforming it into something that is desired but at the same time prohibited and untouchable. Freud states,

> Taboos, we must suppose, are prohibitions of primæval antiquity which were at some time externally imposed upon a generation of primitive men; they must, that is to say, no doubt have been impressed on them violently by the previous generation. These prohibitions must have concerned activities towards which there was a strong inclination.
>
> (Freud 1913: 31)

In his view taboos were passed on from one generation to another via tradition, transmitted via the authority of parents and society and inscribing themselves as unconscious psychic content. In turn, Norbert Elias's theory about the civilizing process held that prohibitions were transmitted unconsciously via the formation of a second social nature or set of habits, leading individuals to repeat unwittingly patterns of behaviour that served the logic of exclusion and distinction of social classes.

"Taboo is a primæval prohibition", Freud states, "forcibly imposed (by some authority) from outside, and directed against the most powerful longings to which human beings are subject" (Freud 1913: 34–35). However, people who are ruled by taboos are ambivalent about them. The desire to transgress the taboo remains in the unconscious:

> In their unconscious there is nothing they would like more than to violate them, but they are afraid to do so; they are afraid precisely because they would like to, and the fear is stronger than the desire. The desire is unconscious, however, in every individual member of the tribe just as it is in neurotics.
>
> (Freud 1913: 31)

The ambivalence of meanings allows the two drives, love and hate, to be directed at the same object. In this sense, Freud is able to conclude that taboos remain in our psychic life for a reason: the desire to make the forbidden continue to exist, as an object of adoration and as a forbidden object.

As we know, Norbert Elias had an in-depth knowledge of Freud's work and, in this sense, it seems no coincidence that he uses the term taboo to refer to the logic that regulates the distancing of the established from the outsiders. As occurred in the small community of Winston Parva, the groups that considered themselves superior tended to exclude marginal groups from their close relationships, creating *contact taboos* around them. As the outsiders were seen as lawless, subversive people, since they did not follow the social restrictions and norms, closer contact with them was perceived as a threat to the cohesion of the established group: "'Inferior' people are apt to break taboos which the 'superior' people have been trained to observe from childhood on" (Elias and Scotson 1965: 153).

In Winston Parva the signs of superiority were inscribed in the members of the group who had been established since their childhood, as they passed from generation to generation. In this sense, the analysis that Elias and Scotson carried out on the stigmatization process of one group over the other via discourses of exaltation and defamation is fundamental. The social cohesion of a group rests on the capacity to create and spread gossip, stigmatizing as inferior the individuals from the excluded zones of Winston Parva. In the case of this small English community, the inhabitants of the oldest zone, who had known each other for a long time and whose families had close contact, were not only more capable of producing gossip, but also needed it to preserve their image as superior beings. According to the authors, the taboo of contact with the outsiders was maintained by means of praise gossip, that referred to members of the established group, and blame gossip, directed at those who had the status of pariahs.

In this way gossip reflects the structure and position of the group where that gossip circulates. The function of gossip was to maintain integration among those similar to each other and to exclude outsiders. Praise gossip served to give value to the person and the group being referred to, highlighting their superiority, their values and their lifestyle. Such gossip exalted their egos, since it reinforced the notion that they were worthy and deserving of their due privileges. It thus represents a discourse that led to a sense of satisfaction for both those who spread it and those who heard it.

Blame gossip had a dual role in setting up the established-outsiders configuration. It served to integrate people who behaved in accordance with norms and requirements, at the same time as excluding those who did not comply with the same moral ideals. However, when negative gossip was spread about other people, it still provoked envy: "And the talk often sounded as if it tickled the imagination of the gossipers to think for a moment that they themselves had done what one should not do" (Elias and Scotson 1965: 93). Fulfilling a prohibited desire provokes envy in those who obey the prohibition as they also have the ability to free themselves from the coercive restrictions imposed on them.

Returning to the significance of the ambivalence in the term contact taboo, as Freud proposes in *Totem and Taboo*, furthers our understanding of the established-outsiders configuration. The outsiders provoke the desire to extricate oneself from the sacrifice of individual freedom, freeing oneself from the social coercions and rules established by tradition. From this perspective, as the following passages illustrate, we can see how Norbert Elias and Sigmund Freud are connected. Together with Scotson, Elias states, "non-observation of their own norms by others is apt to weaken their defence against their own wish to break the prescribed norm" (Elias and Scotson 1965: li). It is better to be free than to be subjected to group obligations, a member of the established group might think. In turn, Freud states, "Anyone who has violated a taboo becomes taboo himself because he possesses the dangerous quality of tempting others to follow his example: why should *he* be allowed to do what is forbidden to others?" (Freud 1913: 32). Those who become similar to outsiders also become taboos.

What is of interest here, stemming from these propositions, is the notion that the logic that Norbert Elias defines as the established-outsiders relationship is not a binary one that separates and isolates the two groups as if they were independent from each other. Rather, what we are dealing with here is a logic of exclusion that cannot be seen as a process of disjunction between the different parts, but as a way of continuously linking one to the other. They are like two versions of the same surface that are continually interlinked with each other. The outsiders are not simply the opposite of the established since they reveal a truth that the established do not want to know about themselves.

3.2 "Us" and "them": questions about identity

The established-outsider configuration confers an excess of power that allows the dominant group to reserve for itself social positions of privilege with much greater potential than the demeaned groups. The established members of Winston Parva, for example, took on the main positions in the community's social institutions, religious associations, clubs, and schools. However, it is not only via economic or material advantages that the established stigmatized those different to them as being inferior. This power imbalance also satisfied other aspirations.

Initially, the recently arrived inhabitants of Winston Parva did not feel different from the long-established residents and therefore tried to become closer to them in some way. However, they ended up being rejected by the long-standing inhabitants, who had built up relationships that were closed to any outsiders that were not part of their histories, or did not share their experiences, memories, and feelings. A common past led to an increase in group cohesion, a high level of identification among its members and the formation of common rules and habits.

Being part of a group, establishing affective ties and identifying with other people, referring to themselves as "us", at the same time as excluding any other individuals who were different as "them", is a process reliant on the creation of identificatory links that involve the coercion of behaviours and feelings. To belong to a group with a high level of cohesion, a price must be paid, and a sacrifice made that demands compensation.

> Participation in a group's superiority and its unique group charisma is, as it were, the reward for submitting to group-specific norms. It has to be paid for by each of its members individually through the subjection of his own conduct to specific patterns of affect control.
>
> (Elias and Scotson 1965: xxiii)

have seen, in Elias's view an individual is never isolated from social relationships. The image that they construct of themselves, their *self-image*, links to the image of the social group they belong to, the *we-image*, whether it is a social class, a social institution, a religion, an ethnicity or a nation. Elias states,

> It is one of the most elementary characteristics of humans that they do not have only an image of themselves as individual persons who can say "I" but also an image of themselves as the members of groups of which they can say "we".
>
> (Elias 1989: 356)

Whether they be British, French, German, or Brazilians, all citizens of a country assimilate particular ways of behaving in accordance with the customs and norms that make them recognize themselves as similar to each other. Elias continues,

> even in highly individualized societies, images of we-group such as the nation belong to the self-image of individuals and that, at the same time, the personality structure of any individual represents one of countless variations on a common national pattern.
>
> (Elias 1989: 356)

Elias called the incorporation of a common code of conduct *habitus*, and he referred to the *self-images* as the *self-ideal* and the *we-images* as the *we-ideal* when people attribute the best values to themselves: "A person's we-image and we-ideal form as much part of a person's self-image and self-ideal as the image and ideal of him – or herself as the unique person to which he or she refers as 'I'" (Elias and Scotson 1965: xliii), conclude the authors in their study of the small English community. When we refer to a specific group that we belong to – stating "I am German", "I am Jewish", or "I am a man", for example –we are declaring that what we are and how we act is in accordance with the identities of this collective entity, repeating the hegemonic patterns instilled and passed on throughout its history. The *we-ideal* of the French provides the parameters for every individual born in France about what their *self-ideal* should be like, namely, what it is to be French, how to behave as a French person, what you can and cannot do to be considered an equal.

This process of imbrication between the changes to social structures and the development of the psychic economy entails antagonism between the narcissistic principles of identification with the identical and the principles of exclusion of alterity. The pride and narcissistic satisfaction in being part of a group that acts in accordance with its ideal stem from the formation process of the *we-image*. At the same time, when we construct a personal image, bearing the marks that insert us into a specific social group, we put ourselves into an antagonistic position in relation to others and we exclude from the sphere of social relationships all those people who have different features.

In this power struggle, the outsiders end up accepting their position as the dominated group, as the "the established groups usually have an ally in an inner voice of their social inferiors" (Elias and Scotson 1965: xxiv). Norbert Elias refers to the superego as a psychic agent that acts not only in a coercive way, but is also recriminatory and punitive, reacting whenever individuals do not manage to attain a given ideal. The outsider groups internalize the derogatory images that the established create of them, as this interior voice, the superego, reproduces their submissive position imposed by those who monopolize the centres of power. From this perspective, those deemed the most inferior evaluate themselves by the standards of their oppressors, reproducing patterns of responses from the position of social detritus: "Give a group a bad name and it is likely to live up to it" (Elias and Scotson 1965: xxviii). The features associated with being "established" or "marginal" are not part of the essence of the group, but particular expressions of behaviour and affect within power relations. It is up to the outsiders and all those in positions of marginality to strive to resist the stigmatizations imposed by the hegemonic groups.

3.3 Intolerances and narcissisms of small differences

When asked about the thinkers who most influenced him during his career, Norbert Elias singled out Freud:

> Among the individual works that have exerted an influence on me, I can really only mention the work of Freud. Freud's psychoanalytic theory has had, as a theory, an important influence on my work. I cannot cite another work, or a specific book that would have had a comparable influence.
>
> (Elias 1987a: 69)

Concepts inherent to psychoanalysis – such as drive, libido, superego, repression, and sublimation – appear to be intrinsically assimilated into the theorization of the civilizing process. The ideas that enabled the formalization of Freud's clinic on the theory of the unconscious interrogate, from their very foundation, the notion of the autonomy of the ego. In his correspondence with his friend Wilhelm Fliess, even before writing his main works, Freud exposed the illusory character of identities, arguing that the ego is a place formed within a set of relationships, whose identifications constitute a "multiplicity of psychic personalities" (Freud 1986: 241). In this sense, in the formation of the ego, the multiple comes to substitute the notion of unity and alterity comes to the fore by revealing itself as an essential element in the formation of the individual. Identity, in Freud's thinking, should be considered as a process that is never completed, made up of a network of identifications whose notions of self are only created in relationship to another.

In Freud's work we can see in the *ego ideal* and the *narcissism of small differences* expressions of ambivalence inherent in all relationships that require the recognition of the other as different at the same time as requiring the elimination of the other because it is a threat. From the perspective, the relationship between the established and the outsiders also contains elements of Freudian metapsychology, recognising the importance of unconscious fantasies and desires in the formation of social configurations: "Humans groups seem to take a strange delight in asserting their superiority over others", writes Elias in *Involvement and Detachment*, "particularly if it has been attained by violent means" (Elias 1983: 16). The ideals of superiority of charismatic groups express narcissistic ideals. At the same time, the differences are reduced to flaws or imperfections that should be kept as far removed as possible. Elias continues,

> The remarkable propensity of people for projecting part of their individual self-love into specific social units, to which they are linked by strong feelings of identity and of belonging, is one of the roots of the dangers which human groups constitute for each other.
>
> (Elias 1983: 17)

The term narcissism exposes not only the impossibility of recognizing the other as alterity, in accordance with the meaning of the expression "self-love", but also intolerance of what presents itself as different. The need to preserve one's identity leaves the ego threatened whenever it comes across something different from itself. In these situations, the immediate response is to distance oneself from these dangerous differences. In Freud's view, rejection of the other is inherent to all human relationships and surfaces in the form of the *narcissism of small differences*. The first time this expression appeared was in the text *The Taboo of Virginity* [*Das Tabu der Virginität*], of 1918, as we see in the following passage:

> Crawley, in language which differs only slightly from the current terminology of psycho-analysis, declares that each in dividual is separated from the others by a "taboo of personal isolation", and that it is precisely the minor differences in people who are otherwise alike that form the basis of feelings of strangeness and hostility between them. It would be tempting to pursue this idea and to derive from this "narcissism of minor differences" the hostility which in every human relation we see fighting successfully against feelings of fellowship and overpowering the commandment that all men should love one another.
>
> (Freud 1918: 199)

When ties are established between people, feelings of estrangement and hostility arise in the face of any trace of differences, despite the points of identification that unite them. Resistance to the proximity of the other outweighs brotherhood, solidarity and altruism, evidencing the fact that when individuals come together, there is a pull away from these principles, which dictate ethical commandments such as "you will love your neighbour as you do yourself". If I love my neighbour, it is because they either resemble me or my ideal of perfection, so I will be able to love them like an ideal of myself. If they are outsiders, why would they be worthy of my love? In this case, Freud says, they would be more deserving of my hate than of any possible love.

The *narcissism of small differences* is taken up again by Freud in the texts *Group Psychology and the Analysis of the Ego* (1921) and *Civilization and Its Discontents* object: the *leader*. Adhering to a common code proves to be like a social insignia. This stimulates the feeling of belonging to the superior group.

What is the mechanism that leads to a group's blind submission to a leader, putting hundreds and thousands of people under the persuasive influence and the power of suggestion of a single individual and creating extreme intolerance of everything not under his influence or subject to the rules he imposes? To answer this question, Freud returns to theories of the libido, of identification and of love.

Identification is a psychic process that links individuals together in a homogeneous unit. Everyone is drawn to a common ideal object, as if the latter were the representative that could transform the ego into the desired model. This is one of the most primordial ways of bringing individuals together, as, via identification, a previously lost narcissistic relationship with those who are similar seeks to be re-established. The individual who is unable to find satisfaction in their own ego resorts to their ideal, the heir of narcissism, which in turn echoes in the collective ideal (*we-ideal*) of the group.

But it is not only a leader that the members of a group identify with. Returning to the theory that Gustave Le Bon puts forward in *The Crowd: A Study of the Popular Mind* (1895), – the roots of which point towards the contractualist thinking of Jean-Jacques Rousseau (1762) about the idea of a *general will* as the will of the sovereign, that body politic that aims for the common good to bring a collective entity together –, Freud states that the leader is given a place of prominence not only due to personal prestige, but also for their ideas, ideas that have fanaticized the leader himself. The sharing of an idea may therefore replace the leader in unifying the members of a group:

> We should consider whether groups with leaders may not be the more primitive and complete, whether in the other an idea, an abstraction, may not take the place of the leader (a state of things to which religious groups, with their invisible head, form a transitional stage), and whether a common tendency, a wish in which a number of people can have a share, may not in the same way serve as a substitute... The leader or the leader idea might also, so to speak, be negative; hatred against a particular person or institution might operate in just the same unifying way, and might call up the same kind of emotional ties as positive attachment.
>
> (Freud 1921: 129–130)

Ambivalent feelings, however, are substrata of identification: "it can turn into an expression of tenderness as easily as into a wish for someone's removal" (Freud 1921: 134), Freud continues. As we know, the text *Group Psychology* was written in the aftermath of major historical events in which large-scale collective entities established the direction of history: the Russian Revolution of 1917, the imperial armies of World War I and, in the 1920s/1930s, the formation of the National Socialist Party in Germany which, as a result of all the horrors and atrocities it committed, gave new meaning to the term "leader" [*die Führer*] with Adolf Hitler's rise to power.

Individuals are formed within collectivities, whose ideals shared by their members are essential for the construction of the ego of each of these individuals. Collectivities unite when a number of individuals identify their ideal in a single object, resulting in the individuals renouncing their *ego-ideals*, replacing them with the group ideal.

> Each individual is a component part of numerous groups, he is bound by ties of identification in many directions, and he has built up his ego ideal upon the most various models. Each individual therefore has a share in numerous group minds – those of his race, of his class, of his creed, of his nationality, etc. – and he can also raise himself above them to the extent of having a scrap of independence and originality.
>
> (Freud 1921: 161)

The participation of an individual in social groups serves to protect them against abandonment, when they find themselves disassociated from any relationship with the other. In this context, it is worth remembering that the feeling of *social fear* or *panic* surfaces when affective ties disappear as a group breaks apart: "It is impossible to doubt that panic means the disintegration of a group; it involves the cessation of all the feelings of consideration which the members of the group otherwise show one another" (Freud 1921: 127). It is preferable to sacrifice an element of individual freedom and submit to the rigorous coercive demands of groups than be faced with the threats of danger when one is alone.

The overlapping between the "I" and the "we" discourses supports Norbert Elias's ideas on the formation of *habitus*, from the process of psychic internalization in the form of a second unconscious nature and from values that permeate a social group. When there is a very small difference between the *self-ideal* and the collective ideal, the sense of triumph at being part of a group with a high level of charisma maintains the child's narcissistic arrogance. The individual thus reproduces and passes on unknowingly through habits, behaviours and emotions, values and ideals that correspond to those of the group they belong to. In exchange for the large amount of love that individuals direct towards the group leader (the representative of the collective ideal) there is a need for them to be recognized and loved by the leader in the same, equitable way.

The interlinking of the *self-ideals* with the *we-ideals* is illustrated, according to Elias's line of thought, in national ideologies and the conviction that the individual has special merit, due to the greatness and superiority of the tradition of their nation. This link establishes particular kinds of *national habitus* that, on the one hand, enable it to unite with members belonging to a common national state, helping them, in this sense, to shut themselves away in a large collectivity when they feel threatened; on the other hand, national ideologies "serve to stoke up the fires of conflict and tension between nations" (Elias 1987d: 82), which is inherent in the ambivalence of the configurations that individuals establish among themselves via the intermediary of national states.

The formation of the *we-identity* based on the organization of society in the form of a state is a recent process, when we consider that majority of its members. If in ancient and absolutist states the "we" referred to a narrow layer of the population, in national states outsiders are those who do not belong to the same nation. Consequently, those who were on the margins could not be considered compatriots, but rather barbarians or pariahs: the *bourgeoisie*, when they were not part of the court; the *workers*, when the bourgeoisie established themselves in control of the state monopoly; the *immigrants*, who do not fit into the group identity of a country's workers, are just a few examples. Conflicts between the established and outsiders, between groups who are "in" and those who are "out", are reproduced in the sense of belonging and identification with the state.

National states, according to Elias, were born from wars and for wars. Sometimes, instead of defending and protecting, they threaten each other and turn on those who do not belong to them or who are outsiders. In this sense, *national habitus* also bear the ambivalence of collective ideals. What enables ties between individuals also leads to distancing between them, says Elias, "Often enough values which represent the essence of what gives life purpose and meaning contribute to the constant renewal of tendencies destructive of life and meaning " (Elias 1987d: 82).

In *Civilization and Its Discontents*, Freud returns to the *narcissism of small differences*, arguing that it is a consequence of the death drive. In the face of impulses or drives, repression transfers erotic, narcissistic and aggressive libidos onto human relationships. Repression of the life drive produces symptoms, whereas repression of the death drive leads to the unconscious feeling of guilt, the destructive effects of which are not weakened even when the individual situates themselves within groups: "the three sources of our suffering: the superior power of nature, the frailty of our bodies, and the inadequacy of the institutions that regulate people's relations with one another in the family, the state and society" (Freud 1930: 86). The difference between *Group Psychology* and *Civilization and Its Discontents* is that the 1930 text see the effects of the death drive consistently in all libidinal ties – even within groups –so it is impossible to avoid the production of suffering.

In the wake of analysis of the Christian commandment "you will love your neighbour as you do yourself", the other, always an outsider, is held up as a receptacle for the discharge of hatred.

> As a result, their neighbour is for them not only a potential helper or sexual object, but also someone who tempts them to satisfy their aggressiveness on him, to exploit his capacity for work without compensation, to use him sexually without his consent, to seize his possession, to humiliate him, to cause him pain, to torture and kill him.
>
> (Freud 1930: 111)

The existence of aggressive tendencies in human relationships is the impossible that makes social ties possible. It is culture's role, in turn, to put limits on hostilities, building identificatory links between individuals. Freud states, with reference to *Group Psychology*,

> I once discussed this phenomenon that it is precisely communities with adjoining territories, and related to each other in other ways as well, who are engaged in constant feuds and in ridiculing each other – like the Spaniards and the Portuguese, the North Germans and the South Germans, the English and the Scots, and so on.
>
> (Freud 1930: 114)

About the *narcissism of small differences*, Freud explains: "We can now see that it is a convenient and relatively harmless satisfaction of the inclination to aggression, by means of which cohesion between the members of the community is made easier" (1930: 114). The *narcissism of small differences*, in this sense, channels this impulse hostility, shifting it onto relationships between individuals. But culture fails even in its aim to sustain illusions.

The *narcissism of small differences* is not only an element of group cohesion. Aggression, Freud states, is part of the substratum of all sentimental relationships between individuals, and thus the other inevitably becomes a target for the destructiveness of the death drive. Aggressions, embedded within human relationships – between individuals, classes, societies and nations –show that the pull towards collectivity leads to the dangerous condition of the "the psychological misery of the mass". Either the intolerance of the *narcissism of small differences* necessitates the *elimination* of the other's difference within the group, or the other is reduced, rejected and stigmatized to the position of social abjects.

References

Elias, Norbert (1950 Dec.) "Studies in the Genesis of the Naval Profession", in *The British Journal of Sociology*, vol. 1, n.4, pp. 291–309.

——— (1969) *The Court Society*. New York: Pantheon Books, 1983.

——— (1970) *What is Sociology?*, trans. by S. Mennell and G. Morrissey. London: Hutchinson & Co, 1978.

——— (1983) *Involvement and Detachment*. Oxford/New York: Basil Blackwell, 1987.

——— (1987a) *J'ai suivi mon propre chemin*. Paris: Les Éditions Sociales, 2016.

——— (1987b) *Norbert Elias: Reflections on a Life*. Cambridge: Polity Press, 1994.

——— (1987c) "Changes in the We-I Balance", in *The Society of Individuals*. London/New York: The Continuum International Publishing Group, 2001.

——— (1987d) "Problems of Self-consciousness and the Image of Man", in *The Society of Individuals*. London/New York: The Continuum International Publishing Group, 2001.

——— (1989) *The Germans. Power Struggles and the Development of Habitus in the Nineteenth and Twentieth Centuries*, trans. by E. Dunning and S. Mennell. New York: Columbia University Press, 1996.

Elias, Norbert and Scotson, John L. (1965) *The Established and the Outsiders – A Sociological Enquiry into Community Problems*. London: Sage Publications, 1994.

Foulkes, Siegmund (1969) "Recollections of My Visit to Freud", in *Selected Papers of S.H. Foulkes: Psychoanalysis and Group Analysis*. London: Karnak Books, 1990.

——— (1971) "The Group as a Matrix of the Individual's Mental Life", in *Selected Papers of S.H. Foulkes: Psychoanalysis and Group Analysis*. London: Karnak Books, 1990.

When Elias places *habitus* at the core of his theory of the civilizing process, pointing out that it is formed through the psychic inscription of self-control mechanisms of drives and affections, he inserts the drive circuit at the base of social structures. For this reason, *habitus* cannot be understood simply as an effect of a learning process, and much less can we see it as a conditioned reproduction of behaviours. In the process of transmission from generation to generation, where instinctual ambivalences are transmitted, *habitus* itself becomes a space for interweaving between individuals and societies, or rather, a condition for the organization of psychic economies circumstantiated by social grammars. Regarding a modern individual, a courtier or someone who lived during feudalism, we must consider not only their differences in relation to social processes, but also in relation to the drive economy of each of them, their psychic elements and their defence mechanisms.

By establishing standards of behaviour, which define what is civilized by the ability to control impulses and emotions, *habitus* function as linking elements between individuals in the same group, as well as being expressions of difference and separation, which can lead to exclusion and annihilation of the other. In more differentiated societies, the layers of *social habitus* that permeate individuals multiply according to the different groups they are part of. Even if the civilizing process goes in the direction of increasing the level of individualization in societies, tending more towards the "I" than towards the "we", not all layers of *social habitus* incline towards this balance. *National habitus* seem to predominate over individual personalities: "Looking more closely", says Elias, "one finds that the traits of national group identity – what we call the 'national character' – are a layer of the social habitus built very deeply and firmly into the personality structure of the individual" (1987b: 209). The histories of states are organized as *national habitus* and are part of the formation of the personality of individuals, with the result that national identity becomes a fundamental element in the construction of people's identity.

With the formation of modern states, the predominance of *national habitus* occurs without difficulties when nations begin to play an increasingly decisive role in people's lives. What was once primarily a social antithesis, such as the German difference between *Kultur* and *Zivilisation,* is re-signified as a national antithesis. Throughout this same process, *national habitus* become central in the construction of the personality of individuals, helping to answer the question "who am I?" through the interweaving of the history of the individual with the history of their state-nation.

One of the functions of the state is to reserve for itself the monopoly of violence and, with this power, serve as a regulator of impulses of aggression and death, whether by individuals, groups or other states. States tend to react to the presence of others, rejecting them and withdrawing into themselves. They end up putting the lives of individuals in danger the moment they feel threatened. In the name of a state's power and sovereignty, lives are lost in wars against enemies inside and outside its own borders. Consequently, an ambivalence is established in the relationship between the state and the individual when, instead of assuming the role of protector and carer, the state itself becomes the executioner.

The "We-I" identity is constructed as memory and relationship, as well as forgetting and segregation. The individual's memory, for instance, is mixed with the memory of his country by remembering and erasing their histories. In this process, the drive circulates with its representatives – emotions and ideas –which in turn suffer the destinies designated by the historical and social processes of each civilization. This is the case for individuals and for nations, as Elias had already identified in *The Civilizing Process* (Elias 1939: 29): "The social units char we call nations differ widely in the affect-economies of their members, in the schemata through which the emotional life of individuals is moulded under the pressure of institutionalized tradition and of the present situation". In different countries and in different historical periods, we see particular civilizing processes that impact on individuals' drive dynamics.

Transmitting the way in which national units build their *self-images*, *national habitus* inscribe in their histories the greatness of their accomplishments and their pride in their ideals, as well as erasing the failure of their defeats and the decadence of their acquisitions. *National habitus*, therefore, have structuring effects to the extent that they can steer the affective identifications of individuals according to their connections with the "we" identity. *National habitus* carry with them the memories of the transformations of states, their continuities and discontinuities, their ruptures and their constructions. Based on the instinctual dynamics of individuals and the formation process of national states, we must think of a psychic economy of *national habitus* whose memory and transmission makes it repeat and reproduce histories of inclusion and segregation, of prejudice and privilege, of rise and fall, of war and peace, of victory and defeat. In Elias's words,

> The French or English person can perhaps tell the German what elements make the concept of civilization the sum of their national self-image. But however reasonable and rational this concept may appear to them, it too grows out of a specific set of historical situations, it too is surrounded by an emotional and traditional aura which is hard to define but wich nevertheless represents an integral part of its meaning. And the discurssion really becomes futile When a German tries to show the French and English person why the concept of *Zivilisation* does indeed represent a value for him, but only one of the second rank.
>
> (1939: 8)

This is the case in Elias's analysis of the civilizing process in France, England, and Germany, for example. Already in *The Civilizing Process* he concluded that concepts such as *civilization* and *culture*, used as a way of distinguishing social classes, also expressed the ways in which each nation built its *self-image*. The imbrication of *national habitus* with feelings and emotions produces fixations and resistance in individuals in relation to changes in their national ideals, leading to the transmission, between generations, of traumas and violence that inflect the direction of the civilizing process towards barbarism and decivilization.

This means, then, that emotions are closely related to the formation of national identities and that these, in turn, participate deeply in the formation of personal identities.

4.2 The duty of memory, a collective responsibility

Norbert Elias was always mindful of the more diverse forms of violence caused by the civilizing process. His research sought to understand how discriminations, segregations, exclusions, wars and acts of barbarism are provoked at the heart of highly civilized groups and societies. Elias also knew the importance of involving people in the traumatic histories that marked societies, especially those that insist on stating: "But we had nothing at all to do with it. Why are we being made responsible for something our fathers did?" (Elias 1989: 429).[1]

After researching the formation of France and England, Norbert Elias lacked an analysis of his own country. Right in the introduction of *The Germans*, he justifies himself. A certain distance was necessary to be able to turn to the German civilizing process and address points that would involve intimate memories of his life that would never cease to be difficult memories. He begins the introduction to the book as follows:

> Standing half-hidden in the background of the studies published here is an eyewitness who has lived for nearly ninety years through the events concerned as they unfolded. The picture of events formed by someone personally affected by them usually differs in characteristic ways from that which takes shape when one views them with the detachment and distance of a researcher.
>
> (Elias 1989: 1)

A little further on he writes,

> Many of the following discussions originated in the attempt to make understandable, to myself and anyone who is prepared to listen, how the rise of National Socialism came about, and thus also the war, concentration camps and the breaking apart of the earlier Germany into two states.
>
> (Elias 1989: 1)

Norbert Elias's sociology is not merely an effort to understand the facts of the past in order to explain present societies. It also encompasses a yearning to bring about changes in the discontent of our civilizations. Right in the introduction to *The Germans*, Elias shows that rescuing memories that were forgotten throughout the formation of societies is the job of sociology when it seeks to bring about transformations in the world. The function of memory then becomes a reparation policy that seeks to restore a commitment by individuals and societies to their repressed histories. Thus, Elias states the following about his work *The Germans*:

> One of the functions of this book is to pave the way intellectually and practically in handling such problems. Perhaps it may have a cathartic effect if the relationship between past and present is seen in this way, and people may, through understanding their social development, find a new understanding of themselves.
>
> (Elias 1989: 19)

We can assume that the idea of a transforming sociology, capable of rebuilding the lost connection between the events repressed by the civilizing process and the formation of our identities, is one of the reasons for the resistance that Elias's work had to face in order to receive its due recognition. It is necessary to question the existence of this silencing, considering that the paradox between marginalization and recognition of Elias's work points to its interpretative power regarding the secrets it reveals about societies, institutions, and individuals, as stated by Paulo Cesar Endo: "But it is likely that an important element in this concealment process is also the insurgent and subversive character that the work contains with regard to the very institutionalization of knowledge and its more or less arbitrary divisions" (2018: 54). A resistance against a work that finds in the heart of social institutions the embryo of the transmission and reproduction of hegemonic patterns of thoughts and behaviour, which establish exclusions and segregations between individuals and social classes.

In the wake of what Hannah Arendt declared in her book *Responsibility and Judgement*, collective responsibility implicates individuals in the process of passing on social traumas. In Arendt's view, responsibility must be differentiated from guilt since it results from the fact that we are all part of a community and that the history of individuals is bound up with the history of society. Arendt writes,

> This vicarious responsibility for things we have not done, this taking upon ourselves the consequences for things we are entirely innocent of, is the price we pay for the fact that we live our lives not by ourselves but among our fellow men.
>
> (Arendt 1968: 157–158)

We cannot be blamed for something that we did not do, but due to the fact that we live collectively, we can assume responsibility for acts committed by others.

Just as Elias contended, Arendt also held that the civilizing process does not destroy acts of violence but passes them on and keeps them alive in the background of public life. In the words of this German philosopher,

> It is in the very nature of things human that every act that has once made its appearance and has been recorded in the history of mankind stays with mankind as a potentiality long after its actuality has become a thing of the past.
>
> (Arendt 1963: 273)

Thinking about future generations, the duty of memory reconstructs the events that have been wiped out, consigned to the crypt of history, so that they will never works were always published with great resistance, and he witnessed the horrors of World War I, in terms of the loss of experience and the silence of the soldiers who returned home. Both lived in Frankfurt during the 1930s and had certain links with the Institute for Social Research. Both fled Germany in 1933, followed by a brief but important stay in Paris, and both were friends of Gisèle Freund. Unlike Elias, who lived for almost a century, Benjamin had a short life, committing suicide at the age of forty in the city of Portbou, Catalonia, while fleeing Nazi persecution.

Elias actually wrote to Benjamin requesting a review of the first volume of *The Civilizing Process*, which had just been published. In the words of Detlev Schöttker (1998), who was responsible for discovering and analyzing the context of this exchange of letters, this review was to have been published in the journal *Zeitschrift für Sozialforshung*, under the editorship of Max Horkheimer, but it never materialized. Not due to lack of interest or disregard for Elias's ideas on the part of Benjamin, who recognized the importance of his work, but above all because he was occupied with his research and involved in his own personal difficulties.

In Benjamin's view, the researcher who turns to the past must consider the interplay of forces produced by class struggles and, therefore, be able to distance himself from the way in which the history of the winners is told by a historiography that aims to link the progress of civilization to the actions of the most powerful. For this form of knowledge, notably a bourgeois and positivist one, he argues that history can be universalized and its truth recovered in all its points of relevance. Benjamin states that the historian must be able to break the *empathy* [*Einfühlun*] with the winners and assume the principle that class struggles have ultimately silenced, repressed, and erased from history those who did not occupy the social positions of power and prestige.

It is necessary, on the contrary, to be an anti-historian, that is, to abandon the pretence of knowing the past as it is in itself, ceasing to write the history of the vanquished in order to be able to rescue the memory of the forgotten, buried by official hegemonic narratives. Consequently, in thesis VII of his text *On the concept of History* [*Über den Begriff der Geschichte*], Benjamin writes,

> Whoever has emerged victorious participates to this day in the triumphal procession in which current rulers step over those who are lying prostrate. According to traditional practice, the spoils are carried in procession. They are called "cultural treasures", and a historical materialist views them with cautious detachment. For in every case these treasures have a lineage which he cannot contemplate without horror. They owe their existence not only to the efforts of the great geniuses who created them, but also to the anonymous toil of others who lived in the same period. There is no document of culture which is not at the same time a document of barbarism. And just as such a document is never free of barbarism, so barbarism taints the manner in which it was transmitted from one hand to another. The historical materialist therefore dissociates himself from this process of transmission as far as possible. He regards it as his task to brush history against the grain.
>
> (1940: 391–392)

The way in which Walter Benjamin understands temporal takes elements from his readings of Freud regarding the functioning of the psychic apparatus, as well as from the psychoanalytic notion of trauma as a disruption of the chronological linearity of events. For Freud, the ruins of the past have not disappeared or been erased but remain active as remnants that have helped us build the present time: "in mental life, nothing that has once taken shape can be lost, that everything is somehow preserved and can be retrieved under the right circumstances", he states in *Civilization and Its Discontents* (Freud 1930: 7). In the view of Freud, Benjamin, and Elias, it seems that the mnemonic materials on which they focus, whether at the psychic, social, or historical level, have been repressed, but continue to be active in the present in a continuous, incomplete, and unfinished temporal flow.

The idea of the fragmentation of time is also important to Benjamin's thinking. For him, the past is present in the course of history as the memory of a dream that soon fades away or a Freudian slip that may not be noticed. As he states, for example, in his work *The Arcades Project* [*Das Passage-Werk*],

> In the dialectical image, what has been within a particular epoch is always, simultaneously, "what has been from time immemorial". As such, however, it is manifest, on each occasion, only to a quite specific epoch – namely, the one in which humanity, rubbing its eyes, recognizes just this particular dream image as such. It is at this moment that the historian takes up, with regard to that image, the task of dream interpretation.
>
> (Benjamin 1982: 464)

As in dreams, where the past is shown to be alive in the present, it is in the encounter between two times that a truth can be revealed. This return to the past, for Benjamin, is driven by an ethical project to rescue a memory that bears witness to the barbarities produced by the civilizing process. Time, in Benjamin's thinking, is the *Now-Time* [*Jetztzeit*], in which the present and the past are interconnected in a strong, potent and explosive way, at the same time that it is a fleeting and fragile connection. A constellation, as the philosopher says, in which you need to have the spirit to be able to grasp the relationship between moments. This encounter with the forgotten events of the past is fundamental so that history can be rewritten, weaving again the threads of experiences that could not be transmitted. There is, therefore, an ethical duty in this remembrance, insofar as it recovers a past that could not be inscribed in the memory of humanity.

Benjamin tries to save from oblivion those excluded from history, those who bring with them the remains of the catastrophe of civilization. It is necessary to brush history against the grain, against the narrative of a so-called official history, seeking out the content that has been erased and forgotten by civilization. It is up to the historiographical researcher to do the same work as refuse workers (Benjamin 1969), who collect the waste thrown away by society, everything that was rejected by the city and cannot remain visible to all. But the civilizing process insists on carrying with it its own ruins, the rubble from the destruction that it brought about over the centuries in an unbridled quest for progress, as Benjamin describes, taking as his reference the painting *Angelus Novus*, by Paul Klee, in his famous thesis IX:

> There is a picture by Klee called *Angelus Novus*. It shows an angel who seems about to move away from something stares at. His eyes are wide, his mouth is open, his wings are spread. This is how the angel of history must look. His face is turned toward the past. Where a chain of events appears before *us*, he sees one single catastrophe, which keeps piling wreckage upon wreckage and hurls it at his feet. The angel would like to stay, awaken the dead, and make whole what has been smashed. But a storm is blowing in from Paradise and has got caught in his wings; it is so strong that the angel can no longer close them. The storm drives him irresistibly into the future, to which his back is turned, while the pile of debris before him grows toward the sky. What we call progress is this storm.
>
> (Benjamin 1940: 392)

This triple relationship between past, present, and future times resurfaces in Benjamin's chosen image, showing that the remains that civilization leaves behind like catastrophes keep piling up to the extent that we do not stop to think about them and inscribe them in our history. The angel of history, this researcher of memories, would like to collect these remains, take care of them, treat the wounds of the victims. However, the future, represented by the desire for progress, forces him increasingly to move forward without looking back. If you do not turn around, you will be destined to repeat the same tragedies endlessly. New catastrophes, new genocides, new acts of exclusion, and violence will continue to bury individuals and societies.

The sense of responsibility poses the need to prevent the resonance of the trauma so that the dark events of the past are not repeated for those yet to come. Like Benjamin, Norbert Elias is personally engaged in this, which was one of his last research projects, taking responsibility for repairing the past to be able to build new histories for those who will follow. It is a task that meets with resistance, as he himself recognizes in the final pages of *The Germans*: "I myself believed for a while that it was time to forget the past" (Elias 1989: 429). However, the experience of having lived through two major wars, losing friends and family in the atrocities committed by the Nazis, was so painful and traumatic that it was time to tackle this creative process.

> Much has been said about coming to terms with the past. But it is quite clear that this has only been repressed and in no way overcome. To speak about it is certainly not easy. I realize that by doing so, one touches an open wound in the we-consciousness of the Germans. But precisely because it has not healed, it is necessary to talk about it – not in order to accuse, but as a prelude to the effort to explain the temporary breakdown of human civilization in Germany. It seems to me that it is important for the health and future of West Germany (if the country does have a future) to draw the problem out of the oblivion into which it has sunk and into the public eye again.
>
> (Elias 1989: 429)

The return of the repressed occurs not only in the intimacy of individual symptoms, but also in the formation of social institutions when the formation of habits and identities brings the social conflicts of past times right into the present. As Elias writes, "For just as in the development of an individual person the experiences of earlier times continue to have an effect in the present, so, too, do earlier experiences in the development of a nation" (1989: 178). The past, in his words, casts its shadow over the present time. It emerges in contemporary narratives in a violent way, forcing the repetition of a path that has already been trodden, no longer as a memory, since it has been forgotten, but now as an act.

In the text *Remembering, Repeating and Working-Through* [*Erinnern, Wiederholen und Durcharbeiten*], written by Freud in 1914, the term working-through [*Durcharbeiten*] is presented as a fundamental technique for anyone conducting psychoanalysis, distinguishing its clinical practice from all the therapies that use the method of suggestion. In the early days of his clinic, as documented in his *Studies on Hysteria* [*Studien über Hysterie*] (Freud and Breuer 1895), Freud used hypnosis to recall the causes of hysterical symptoms. At that point, suspending resistance to the memory of traumatic events was enough to produce a first step in healing, since, as he stated at the time, all hysterics suffer from reminiscences. Gradually, with the development of clinical and theoretical work, he recognized that even under the influence of hypnosis, some unconscious resistance prevented the memory of pathogenic representations. This therefore led to the formation of defence psychoneuroses (obsessional neurosis, hysteria, phobia, and paranoia) as psychoanalytic psychic structures. Gradually, hypnosis was replaced by the free association rule, whose therapeutic effects were produced in the transferential relationship between patient and psychoanalyst. From that moment on, it was up to the psychoanalyst to find the associative ties between the memories that patients recounted about their lives. Both techniques, Freud writes, retained a common denominator of psychoanalytic treatment: "Descriptively speaking, it is to fill in gaps in memory; dynamically speaking, it is to overcome resistances due to repression" (Freud 1914: 148).

In 1905, the Spanish poet and essayist George Santayana wrote in his book of poems *The Life of Reason*: "Those who cannot remember the past are condemned to repeat it" (1905: 82). Art again anticipated what psychoanalysis later concluded with the formulation of the concept of repetition compulsion. In this text from 1914, Freud points out that certain experiences that are part of the beginnings of childhood, and whose contents the child would not have the psychological conditions to remember, end up reappearing not in the form of a memory, but repeated as an act:

> the patient does not *remember* anything of what he has forgotten and repressed, but *acts* it out. He reproduces it not as a memory but as an action; he *repeats* it, without, of course, knowing that he is repeating it.
>
> (Freud 1914: 150)

This occurs in the process of psychoanalytic treatment, when, for example, the patient who does not remember having been stubborn and rebellious with their parents reproduces the same behaviour in their relationship with the analyst. The repetition of memories that are difficult to remember is not limited to the treatment context but is acted out in individuals' most diverse relationships. Furthermore, as Freud points out, the recognition of traumatic histories becomes a practice so that the past does not repeat itself in the form of an act. In his words,

> His illness itself must no longer seem to him contemptible, but must become an enemy worthy of his mettle, a piece of his personality, which has solid ground for its existence and out of which things of value for his future life have to be derived. The way it thus paved from the beginning for a reconciliation with the repressed material which is coming to expression. In his symptoms, while at the time place is found for a certain tolerance for the state of being ill.
>
> (Freud 1914: 150)

The idea that the therapeutic process works by reconstructing lost memories was already present in the early days of psychoanalytic theory and technique, and consequently on several occasions the comparison between the work of psychoanalysts and that of archaeologists served as an analogy. In the same way that the ruins of civilization appear to archaeologists through the recovery of materials buried by time, psychoanalysis is also concerned with material forgotten in the unconscious. According to the specificity of psychoanalytic archaeology, it is possible to state that at the root of neurotic symptoms, at the foundation of civilization and within the discontent of culture, repression operates on drives, leaving vestiges that remain active in the unconscious. Thus, both the archaeologist and the psychoanalyst have the same task of accessing lost material and filling in gaps in memory through the process of building their histories. However, unlike the ruins of civilizations, psychic material is not destroyed by repression. It remains timelessly conserved in the unconscious, from where it returns in the form of symptoms, dreams, or repetitions.

4.3 The construction of cases: Norbert Elias's Mozart

Freud draws many comparisons between psychoanalytical work and that of archaeologists, as we see in the text *Constructions in Analysis* [*Konstruktionen in der Analyse*], of 1937. In this work, *construction* is presented as an elaboration technique that seeks to fill the gaps in a patient's memory, recovering material that has been repressed and cannot be accessed. Freud states,

> His work of construction, or, if it is preferred, of reconstruction, resembles to a great extent an archaeologist's excavation of some, dwelling-place that has been destroyed and buried or of some ancient edifice, The two processes are in fact identical, except that the analyst works under better conditions and has more material at his command to assist him, since what he is dealing with is not something destroyed but something that is still alive, and perhaps for

> another reason as well. But just as the archaeologist builds up the walls of the building from the foundations that have remained standing, determines the number and position of the columns from depressions in the floor and reconstructs the mural decorations and paintings from the remains found in the debris, so does the analyst proceed when he draws his inferences from the fragments of memories, from the associations and from the behaviour of the subject of the analysis. Both of them have an undisputed right to reconstruct by means of supplementing and combining the surviving remains.
>
> (Freud 1937b: 259)

The purpose of analytical work is to remember certain experiences that were forgotten due to the force of repression and that, still active, produce symptoms as substitutes for what was forgotten. To recover forgotten memories, remnants become traces that the psychoanalyst can work with: dream fragments, memories that arise through free association, symptomatic formations, or repetitions of behaviours in the transference relationship. It is psychoanalyst's job to build the associative links between these memory traces, retrieving a part of his patient's lost history. The technique of psychoanalysis, therefore, rather than proposing an interpretation, is based on the method of construction in analysis:

> "Interpretation" applies to something that one does to some single element of the material, such as an association or a parapraxis. But it is a "construction" when one lays before the subject of the analysis a piece of his early history that he has forgotten, in some such way as this: "Up to your nth year you regarded yourself as the sole and unlimited possessor of your mother; then came another baby and brought you grave disillusionment. Your mother left you for some time, and even after her reappearance she was never again devoted to you exclusively. Your feelings towards your mother became ambivalent, your father gained a new importance for you",... and so on.
>
> (Freud 1937b: 261)

The analogy between the work of the archaeologist and that of the psychoanalyst also extends to Norbert Elias's sociological research method, whereby he proposes to construct the history of the formation of modern states from fragments, remnants of memories, apparently minor elements that were forgotten or repressed by the civilizing process, but that remain and are active in the formation of the discontent of our civilization. Elias also analyzes the tensions, flaws, and ruptures that permeate different social configurations. In this sense, Freud's and Elias's objects of study are similar because by not limiting themselves to discussing ideas and great theories, nor to investigating major social revolutions, they focus on the most obscure aspects of the psychopathology of everyday life, which are therefore not easily understood by any researcher.

What are the origins and purposes of our dreams, our symptoms, and our habits? How do we construct our individual and collective identities? These are some of the questions that both Freud and Elias asked themselves from the beginning of their research, and that led them to investigate elements that until then had not been explained by any other researcher. If Freud showed us that individuals manifest their neuroses through their symptoms and that these are nothing more than repetitions of histories whose origins are unknown to them, Elias was able to identify, in the formation of *habitus* and customs, repetitions within the civilizing process whose origins and intentions are unknown to individuals and societies.

It is the role of the psychoanalyst to reveal a truth that emerges from constructing the history of individuals from the unelaborated vestiges of their past, as is illustrated in this passage from Freud:

> That work would consist in liberating the fragment of historical truth from its distortions and its attachments to the actual present day and in leading it back to the point in the past to which it belongs. The transposing of material from a forgotten past on to the present or on to an expectation of the future is indeed a habitual occurrence in neurotics no less than in psychotics.
>
> (Freud 1937b: 268)

It is also the role of sociological research to rescue, within the civilizing process, the remnants of past times that remained forgotten, but which constitute a truth to be revealed, as Freud continues:

> If we consider mankind as a whole and substitute it for the single human individual, we discover that it too has developed. delusions which are inaccessible to logical criticism and which contradict reality. If, in spite of this, they are able to exert an extraordinary power over men, investigation leads us to the same explanation as in the case of the single individual. They owe their power to the element of historical truth which they have brought up from the repression of the forgotten and primaeval past.
>
> (Freud 1937b: 269)

Norbert Elias sought to elucidate the formation process of great nations, and he was unconcerned with the importance of great historical personalities, unless it was to consider them within the power games inherent in the relationships of interdependence of the social configurations which they were part of. This position, however, did not prevent him from returning to the life and work of Wolfgang Amadeus Mozart to understand how the transformations of societies affect the dynamics and psychic economy of individuals.

Elias's studies on the life of the German musicians, brought together by the editor Michael Schröter in the book *Mozart: Portrait of a Genius* [*Mozart, Zur Soziologie eines Genies*], do not intend to be a biography that isolates an individual's actions from their social relations. Quite the reverse. The analyses he carried out, especially regarding Mozart's correspondence with friends and family, are constructions[2] based on a life trajectory that can only be understood by considering the places of exclusion and belonging within a society undergoing profound transformation. In this sense, Elias's constructions must be placed within a propositional ethics, framing his sociology as a science that aims to bring about transformations in individuals and societies, as we see in a footnote to *Mozart*:

> Sociology is usually regarded as a destructive, reductive discipline. I do not share this view. For me sociology is a science that ought to help us understand better, and explain, what is incomprehensible in our social life. This is why I have chosen the seemingly paradoxical subtitle "The sociology of a genius". It is not my purpose to destroy genius or reduce it to something else, but to make its human situation easier to understand, and perhaps help in some small way to answer the question of what should be done to prevent a fate like Mozart's from happening. By presenting his tragedy as I try to do – and it is only an example of a more general problem – it may be possible to make people more aware of the need to behave more considerately towards innovators.
>
> (Elias 1991: 14)

Elias's work on Mozart, therefore, is not only a study of that enigmatic personality, in a context of transition between court society and the German bourgeoisie in the 18th century, but also a proposal for a transforming sociology that by retrieving the forgotten past, seeks to break with the compulsion to repeat it in the future. The thesis on which Norbert Elias builds his studies on Mozart's life and work is based on his work on the configuration of established groups and outsider groups, placing the Austrian musician as an outsider within a society that because it is constituted on closed codes and with little mobility, failed to recognize his creative abilities or accept his musical genius. The subjective effects on the individual who occupies the place of an outsider and at the same time feels equal or superior to the members of the established group end up intensifying the desire to be recognized as a peer, to be accepted and to be treated as an equal. Consequently, right at the start of *Mozart*, in the section "He Simply Gave Up and Let Go", Elias puts forward his theory about what might have led the musician to a premature death at the age of 35:

> The word "tragedy" may sound somewhat platitudinous and grandiose in this connection. Nevertheless, it can be said with some justice that the tragic side of Mozart's existence was that he, who had striven so hard to win people's love, should have felt while still young, as he did at the end of his life, that he was no longer loved by anyone, not even himself. That is undoubtedly the kind of meaninglessness that someone can die of. At the end, it seems, Mozart was in a state of loneliness and despair. He really knew that he was soon to die, and in his case that must have meant that he also wished to die, and that in large measure he wrote the Requiem for himself.
>
> (Elias 1991: 5–6)

Mozart felt like an outsider his whole life. As was the case in the entire European court, standards of behaviour and tastes were established by the aristocracy and extended to all classes as values and ideals to be assimilated and reproduced.

> desire to be loved, detectable as a dominant wish throughout his life, very largely determined what had meaning for him and what did not. As a child he needed constant reassurance that he was loved, and if this need went unsatisfied he openly showed his sadness and despair.
>
> (Elias 1991: 68–69)

In the biography of Mozart written by Henry-Marie Beyle, better known as Stendhal (1991), the author of *The Red and the Black*, there is a curious passage from his childhood. Always very dependent on the love of others, he repeatedly asked people who were close to him: do you like me? When he got no for an answer, he immediately burst into tears. This was a condition that lasted throughout his life, as Elias describes:

> As a grown man he was hardly less sensitive and vulnerable. The search for proofs of love, for friendship and affection, behind which one senses a measure of self-hate, a feeling of not being lovable, remained one of his dominant traits.
>
> (1991: 69)

The importance of the *we-image* in the formation of the *self-image* permeates the relationship between Mozart, his father, and the society of his time. Leopold Mozart came from a family of artisans. He was able to rise socially because of his musical background, finding a place among the Salzburg aristocracy as a substitute conductor. But this was not enough to place him in a better position than that of a court official. The recognition of his son as a premature genius may have awakened in his father the desire to reach a higher social position, which he himself had not achieved through his own efforts.

Elias's "diagnostic hypothesis", as he himself refers to his interpretation, is as follows: "There is therefore good reason to say that Leopold Mozart tried to achieve the previously absent fulfilment of his life through his son" (Elias 1991: 70). What Mozart's father projected onto his son as a way of rising through the social hierarchy, "found a response in the strong need for love of the child, to whom the musical stimulus from his father clearly gave pleasure", writes Elias (1991: 74). The father's desire to find a meaning for his life in belonging to court society impacted on his son as a demand for love and recognition. But in order to break free from paternal demands, it was also necessary to free himself from the constraints established by court society.

The psychoanalytic concept of "construction in analysis" refers to the moment in which the psychoanalyst comes up with a supplement for the gaps in the memories that the patient cannot remember. To do so, it is necessary to see the individual within a network of interdependent relationships that permeate all levels of their life, from the family, where the first experiences take place and where the first personality traits are formed, to the most complex configurations, such as social classes, religious communities, and the state. In the context of analyses of Wolfgang Amadeus Mozart's memoirs, Norbert Elias precisely situates how the musical prodigy's process of subjective formation was intrinsically intertwined with the way he inserted himself in the transformation process of social classes. Changes in the dynamics and economy of psychic structures are thus intimately linked with changes in the structures of society. As Elias shows us, Mozart's society was undergoing profound transformations. For this reason, the life of the Austrian musician reappears in the first section of the first chapter of *The Germans*, entitled "Civilization and Informalization", to help think about the changes in European patterns of behaviour in the 20th century.

One of the main factors of these transformations concerns the interweaving between established groups and outsider groups, breaking with the crystallization of social barriers. It was possible to find in Mozart, that individual who lived between two worlds, both a formal and an informal style of social behaviour for individuals from higher and lower strata respectively. Elias writes,

> The society of Mozart's time was thus characterized simultaneously by a formality in contact between people of socially higher and lower standing which in its ceremonial severity far exceeded any corresponding formality of our times, and an informality within one's own group which likewise far exceeded what is now possible in social intercourse with people of relatively equal status.
>
> (1989: 28)

What is at issue in the analyses of the informalization spurt are reductions in the power differential between men and women, between parents and children, between colonizing and colonized countries, and between rulers and ruled. Now, if the theory of the civilizing process maintains that, over the centuries, there have been changes in behaviour controls, reducing the strength of external coercion and increasing the mechanisms of individual self-coercion, how are we to understand the loosening of behavioural regulation in this drive towards informalization? Are we living in a time of civilization's retreat towards barbarism? Can Norbert Elias's theory on the civilizing process still explain the transformations of social behaviour in a given period of time? These questions, posed by Elias himself in his book *The Germans*, serve to show how when customs become more flexible this can, in certain situations, mean a reversal of the civilizing process, but does not necessarily impede or even eliminate its trajectory.

The informalization of behaviour does not mean a decivilizing retreat, but a controlled relaxation of self-regulation mechanisms. Those who accuse Norbert Elias of arguing that social transformations move from more permissive to more prohibitive relationships ultimately do not understand the function of coercion. It is certainly not a matter of thinking that the path of civilization tends towards the formation of elements of self-control marked by a search for autonomy, such as obedience to subjective principles as in the Kantian categorical imperative. If this hypothesis was constructed philosophically, it is because it expresses a courtly morality of self-control, the aim of which is independence from external constraints and the distancing of drives and emotions. Elias was very aware of this problem and therefore linked the economy of the unconscious to social processes. Like Freud, he inscribed the dynamics of drives within social processes, which implies the impossibility of all sorts of control and rationality. Behind the movements of civilizing processes, we find a circuit of drives that follows not only the *associative path*, establishing links, approximations and convergences, but also the *dissociative path*, which causes ruptures, disjunctions, and regressions.

What is fundamental, therefore, is to understand that the nature of civilizing processes is that they follow a course wherein the balance between external social constraints and individual self-coercions changes. Consequently, over time, the processes of self-coercion become stronger than those of external coercion. However, it should always be emphasized that regardless of the predominance of external constraints [*Fremdzwänge*] or self-constraints [*Selbstkontrolle*], there is always a return of the repressed that is repeated as a discontent of civilization or as an individual neurosis.

> Let us consider a child who is often hit by its angry father whenever, in his view, it has been naughty. Such a child will learn to avoid disapproved behaviour out of fear of its father. But its self-constraint apparatus will in this respect develop only partially. In order to be able to restrain itself, it remains dependent on others' threats. Its capacity to restrain itself could develop more strongly if the father were to make the child avoid the disapproved behaviour of its own accord, through persuasion, reasoning and signs of caring. But the child who is often hit does not learn to restrain itself independently of an external constraint, without the threat of paternal punishment, and is accordingly also to a great extent at the mercy of its own impulses of hatred and hostility. It is highly probable that such a child will in turn become a beater, taking the father as a model without knowing it.
>
> (Elias 1989: 33–34)

Certain memories, prevented from being remembered, end up being recalled in the form of an act. Norbert Elias thus goes on to draw a correlation between the child's state of dependence on their parent and political systems:

> Members of a state-society which has long been absolutist – ruled from above in the form of what we would call a police state – develop quite analogous personality structures, in which their ability to exercise self constraint remains dependent on an external constraint, on a strong force which threatens them with punishment from outside. A non-absolutist, multi-party regime requires a far stronger and firmer apparatus of self-constraint.
>
> (Elias 1989: 34)

More than an analogy between what happens at the level of individual relations and what happens at the level of social relations, what we see is a process of imbrication between the formation of states and the psychic economy of individuals.

Identified with the figure of a strong and authoritarian leader, the German State does not facilitate the construction of self-regulating psychic mechanisms. Forms of identity politics typical of absolutist, dictatorial, or totalitarian systems, by providing protection and security, create individuals dependent on a greater power whose strength and violence subjugates them and threatens them with rigid norms. In this way, a violent father is taken as a model of authority by the son to the extent that he also constructs his identity on the basis of an authoritarian state that obliges him, via the power of coercion, to obey its leaders as absolute representatives of power and to rely on this political thinking to tell himself what he can do or what he can want. Totalitarian governments engender relationships between individuals that are sustained by the *passion for servitude* without, however, assuming responsibility for the psychological and political consequences of this logic of submission.

Notes

1 Elias, Norbert (1989) *The Germans. Power Struggles and the Development of Habitus in the Nineteenth and Twentieth Centuries*, trans. by E. Dunning and S. Mennell. New York: Columbia University Press, 1996, p. 429.

2 For anyone who thinks that the use of the *construction in analysis* technique does not apply to a topic or even to an individual who they have not had personal knowledge of, who is not a patient, or who has died a long time ago, we only need to recall Freud's work *Delusion and Dreams in Jensen's Gradiva*. Originally published in 1907, Freud takes up the work *Gradiva* (1903) by Wilhelm Jensen in which the author tells the story of a young archaeologist who, in the quest to unearth his history and his past, dedicates his entire life to the study of the ruins of Pompeii after coming across the image of Gradiva in a museum of Roman antiquities. In the construction that stems from dreams, childhood memories and fantasies of Jensen's character, Freud concludes that psychic material is not destroyed by the force of repression but remains conserved in the unconscious in a timeless way, returning to the subject in the guise of symptoms or dreams. The forgetting of a memory presupposes a re-encounter with its lost object.

3 The use of the terms *Kultur* and *Zivilisation* in the formation of the German state was thoroughly dissected by Elias in the first volume of his work *The Civilizing Process* and is dealt with in the second chapter of this book: "Whereas the concept of civilization has the function of giving expression to the continuously expansionist tendency of colonizing groups, the concept of *Kultur* mirrors the self-consciousness of a nation which had constantly to seek out and constitute its boundaries anew, in a political as well as a spiritual sense, and again and again had to ask itself: 'What really is our identity?'" (Elias 1939: 7).

References

Arendt, Hannah (1963) *Eichmann in Jerusalem. A Report on the Banality of Evil*. New York: Penguin Books, 2006.

——— (1968) *Responsibility and Judgment*, ed. by J. Kohn. New York: Schoken Books, 2003.

Bauman, Zigmunt (1979) "The Phenomenon of Norbert Elias", in *Sociology*, vol. 13, n.1, pp. 117–125. www.jstor.org/stable/42852071.

——— (1989) *Modernity and the Holocaust*. New York: Cornell University Press, 2000.

Benjamin, Walter (1940) "On the Concept of History", in *Walter Benjamin: Selected Writings, vol. 4: 1938–1940*, ed. by H. Eiland and M. Jennings. Cambridge, MA: Harvard University Press, 2012.

——— (1969) *Charles Baudelaire: A Lyric Poet in the Era of High Capitalism*, trans. by H. Zohn. London/New York: Verso, 1997.

——— (1982) *The Arcades Project*, trans. by H. Eiland and K. McLaughlin. Cambridge, MA: Harvard University Press, 1999.

Dunning, Eric and Mennell, Stephen (1979) "Figurational Sociology: Some Critical Comments on Zygmunt Bauman's, 'The Phenomenon of Norbert Elias'", in *Sociology*, vol. 13, n.3, pp. 497–501. www.jstor.org/stable/42853383.

Elias, Norbert (1939) *The Civilizing Process. Sociogenetic and Psychogenetic Investigations*, ed. by E. Dunning, J. Goudsblom and S. Mennell, trans. by E. Jephcott. Oxford: Blackwell Publishing, 2013.

——— (1969) *The Court Society*. New York: Pantheon Books, 1983.

——— (1985) "Continuités et discontinuités dans la transmission du savoir", in *La dynamique sociale de la conscience. Sociologie de la connaissance et des sciences*, ed. by Norbert Elias. Paris: La Découverte, 2016.

——— (1987a) *J'ai suivi mon propre chemin: un parcours dans le siècle*. Paris: Les Éditions Sociales, 2016.

——— (1987b) "Changes in the We-I Balance", in *The Society of Individuals*, ed. by Norbert Elias. London/New York: The Continuum International Publishing Group, 2001.

——— (1989) *The Germans. Power Struggles and the Development of Habitus in the Nineteenth and Twentieth Centuries*, trans. by E. Dunning and S. Mennell. New York: Columbia University Press, 1996.

——— (1991) *Mozart: Portrait of a Genius*, ed. by M. Schöter, trans. by E. Jephcott. Cambridge: Polity Press, 1993.

Elias, Norbert and Scotson, John L. (1965) *The Established and the Outsiders – A Sociological Enquiry into Community Problems*. London: Sage Publications, 1994.

Endo, Paulo Cesar (2018) "A incidência do pensamento de Sigmund Freud na obra de Norbert Elias e a radicalidade no exame dos processos civilizadores", in *Psicanálise e Teoria Política Contemporânea*, ed. by A. Costa, G. Costardi and P. Endo. São Paulo: Annablume.

Freud, Sigmund (1914) "Remembering, Repeating and Working-Through", in *The Standard Edition of the Complete Psychological Works of Sigmund Freud – XXX (1911–1913)*, vol. XII, ed. and trans. by J. Strachey. London: The Hogarth Press, 1981.

——— (1930) "Civilization and Its Discontents", in *The Standard Edition of the Complete Psychological Works of Sigmund Freud – The Future of an Illusion, Civilization and its Discontents and Other Works (1927–1931)*, vol. XXI, ed. and trans. by J. Strachey. London: The Hogarth Press, 1981.

——— (1937a) "Analysis Terminable and Interminable", in *The Standard Edition of the Complete Psychological Works of Sigmund Freud – Moses and Monotheism, An Outline of Psycho-analysis and Other Works (1937–1939)*, vol. XXIII, ed. and trans. by J. Strachey. London: The Hogarth Press, 1981.

——— (1937b) "Constructions in Analysis", in *The Standard Edition of the Complete Psychological Works of Sigmund Freud – Moses and Monotheism, An Outline of Psychoanalysis and Other Works (1937–1939)*, vol. XXIII, ed. and trans. by J. Strachey. London: The Hogarth Press, 1981.

Freud, Sigmund and Breuer, Joseph (1895) "Studies on Hysteria", in *The Standard Edition of the Complete Psychological Works of Sigmund Freud – Studies on Hysteria (1893–1895)*, vol. II, ed. and trans. by J. Strachey. London: The Hogarth Press, 1981.

Mennell, Stephen (2001) "The Other Side of the Coin: Decivilizing Processes", in *Norbert Elias and Human Interdependencies*, ed. by T. Salumets. Québec: McGill-Queen's University Press.
Santayana, George (1905) *The Life of Reason or the Phase of Human Progress, Vol. 1 – Reason in Common Sense*. New York: Charles Scribner's Sons, 1953.
Schöttker, Detlev (1998) "Norbert Elia and Walter Benjamin: An Exchange of Letters and its Context", in *History of the Human Sciences*, vol. 11, n.2, pp. 45–59.
Stendhal (1991) *The Life of Mozart*, trans. by D. Sloate. Montreal: Guernica.

balance increasingly swings towards the former. In his work *The Germans*, Elias would go on to describe the most perilous effects brought on by the swinging of *this* pendulum. Contrary to the notion that civilization should be understood as completed and finalized, he insists that the civilizing process does not move in a single direction, but rather takes the form of steps forward and steps back caused by civilizing and decivilizing forces that can occur simultaneously in certain societies. Elias then draws our attention to the fact that no civilization is protected against potential collapse:

> The civilization of which I speak is never completed and always endangered. It is endangered because the safeguarding of more civilized standards of behaviour and feeling in society depends on specific conditions. One of these is the exercise of relatively stable self-discipline by the individual person. This, in turn, is linked to specific social structures. These include the supply of goods – that is, the maintenance of the accustomed standard of living. They also include above all the peaceful solving of intra-state conflicts – that is, social pacification. But the internal pacification of a society, too, is always endangered. It is endangered by social as well as personal conflicts, which are normal attributes of human communal living – the very conflicts which the pacifying institutions are concerned with mastering.
>
> (Elias 1989: 173)

Norbert Elias never deviated from one of his main objectives, which was to establish a close link between the structuring of society and the structuring of personality. In a relationship of difference that is not disconnected, individuals and societies cannot be considered separate entities, isolated, autonomous or independent of each other. The structure that regulates the dynamics and psychic economy of individuals is closely bound up with the structure that underpins social structures, whether in the field of relationships between groups, classes, or institutions, as well as in that of modern states and their inter-state relations. This argument gives rise to the idea that the mechanisms of self-control are structured in accordance with the political models of government – authoritarian or parliamentary democracies, for example – by means of identifications that articulate the image that individuals create of themselves, as collective or individual entities. Between the psychic economy and the social grammar, we find a relationship of mutual determination.

As we will see below, despite Norbert Elias not using the notion of trauma as a fundamental concept to explain the formation process of the *habitus* of German in the 19th and 20th centuries, this did not prevent the term from recurrently appearing and taking on a degree of importance in the work *The Germans*, dialoguing with some elaborations of Freudian theory about trauma. Elias also does not fail to consider the circulation of emotions that permeate the correlative processes of the formation of the personalities of individuals and social institutions. The image that every individual has of themselves, their *self-image*, is constructed on the basis of identification with the image that the group to which they belong transmits to its member, the *we-image*. Bound up with a dose of narcissism that imposes itself on the relationship between an individual and society, these images end up taking the form of the *self-ideal* and, collectively, they take the form of the *we-ideal*. Thus, the history of the group, social class, or nation-state is also bound up with the personal history of each individual.

5.1 Considerations on times of war and trauma

The concept of violence has always been fundamental in the work of both Norbert Elias and Sigmund Freud. Both pored over the subject at different points in their work, but even so many authors end up criticizing them for the way they dealt with the theme of violence in their thinking. Elias was – and still is – devalued for not having given due emphasis to violence in this theorization, concentrating more on pacification as the direction pursued by the civilizing process. Critics of Freud, in turn, focus on the fact that he did not approach violence from the starting point of social processes, especially with regard to the political and economic models of social organization, concentrating more on violence as part of the unconscious activity and experience of the individual, whether in terms of sexual or deadly violence or as the inevitable discontents of relationships with the other.

Norbert Elias and Sigmund Freud, however, were men who lived through dark times and each in his own way was able to interrogate himself about violence as it affected his own personal life. Freud lived through World War I, but he did not live to witness the horrors of the Second. He died in London on 23 September 1939, after being obliged to leave Vienna, the city where he had spent most of his life, as well as four of his sisters, who later died in Nazi concentration camps. Given his advanced age – he was almost 60 – he was not called up to fight in World War I. This does not mean that he did not personally experience the violence of that period, since many of his family member, as well as psychoanalysts that he was close to, did not share his luck. In terms of his children, Jean-Martin volunteered in August 1914, going to serve in the army in Galicia, Russia, and Italy. Oliver was recruited as an engineer, whereas Ernst ended up fighting in Italy from April 1915. Of his closest psychoanalyst colleagues, Max Eitingon fought in the Austrian army as a surgeon in Prague and Hungary, while Karl Abraham also served as a surgeon in east Prussia. Otto Rank was in the heavy artillery in Krakow, and Sándor Ferenczi served as a doctor in Budapest and later as a psychiatrist in a military hospital.

The war that took place mobilized the deepest emotions in every human being, especially those feelings that related to everybody's nationalistic traits. Freud, who had never identified as an Austrian citizen or with the city of Vienna, declared to his friend, the psychoanalyst Karl Abraham on 26 July 1914:

> However, perhaps for the first time in 30 years I feel myself to be an Austrian and would like to try it once again with this not very hopeful Empire. Morale everywhere is excellent. The liberating effect of the courageous action and the secure prop of Germany contribute a great deal to this.
>
> (Freud 2002: 575)

The following month Freud seemed quite confident about German's declaration of war against Belgium, France and Great Britain, writing to Sándor Ferenczi on 23 August 1914:

> The rush of enthusiasm in Austria swept me along with it, at first. In place of well-being and the international practice, which have long since dissipated, I hoped to get a viable fatherland from which the storm of war had wafted away the worst miasmas and in which the children could live with confidence. Like many others, I suddenly mobilized libido for Austria-Hungary.
>
> (Freud 1996: 13)

Freud's enthusiasm for the war gradually turned into a sense of disappointment with the withdrawal of Austro-Hungarian troops from Serbia. His hope, at that point, still lay in the hands of the Germans. He believed in Germany's victory over the Allies, recognizing the sense of nationalistic pride that this would lead to among the German people upon defeating their enemies. "One won't be able to go to England for a long time after the war. Who knows whether to Italy? Germany will also be impossible, in consequence of the Germans' not unjustified arrogance" (Freud 1996: 14). However, things were not going so well in the Freud household. As the war progressed it led to a sense of absence and lack. The absence of his children, of his colleagues, of his patient, a lack of heating and a lack of food. Freud's practice experienced a drastic decline. After the summer holidays he was seeing only one or two patients per week, which by the end of the first year of war did not even amount to six sessions a week.

The absence of his psychoanalyst colleagues, the suspension of the meetings of the Vienna Psychoanalytic Society and the cancellations of the Congresses of the IPA (*International Psychoanalytical Association*), left Freud very solitary in the psychoanalytical world. Furthermore, his optimism about the German army was also beginning to negatively affect his personal friendships. From the other side of Europe, Ernest Jones, the young English psychoanalyst who was to be become one of those most responsible for ensuring his exile on the eve of World War II, had given hope that psychoanalysis would expand its territory beyond the Jewish and German-speaking community. In war time, even simple correspondence between enemy countries was suspended, had to be deviated via another route or took days to arrive. "None of us has news of Jones, I take it? Do you also find it such a strange feeling that he belongs to our 'enemies'?" (Freud 2002: 594), Freud asked Abraham. His short-lived nationalism thus verged on doing on what only a war is able to do, namely to equate foreigners with enemies.

Throughout this period, Freud had already abandoned the hope that the war would contribute something to civilization. In a letter to his female friend Lou Andreas-Salomé, of 25 November 1914, he wrote:

> I do not doubt that mankind will survive even this war, but I know for certain that for me and my contemporaries the world will never again be a happy place. It is too hideous. And the saddest thing about it is that it is exactly

> the way we should have expected people to behave from our knowledge of psycho-analysis. Because of this attitude to mankind I have never been able to agree with your blithe optimism. My secret conclusion has always been: since we can only regard the highest present civilization as burdened with an enormous hypocrisy, it follows that we are organically unfitted for it.
>
> (Freud 1972: 21)

Unlike Freud, Norbert Elias experienced the two great wars of the 20th century. At the age of 18 he took part in World War I, after six months of training in the Soviet Union. During World War II he was obliged to go into exile in England, was detained in an English concentration camp, on the Isle of Man, and lost his mother who was murdered by the Nazis in a concentration camp. He also witnessed the long trajectory of the Cold War and the threat of the outbreak of a nuclear war, but he died before knowing its outcome. Although the topic of violence was not directly discussed in any of his works, we can recognize, however, that *The Civilizing Process*, as a reflection on the psychic mechanisms controlling violence, that *The Germans*, in its discussion of violence in the *habitus* of the German people and the historical events that formed part of Germany's civilizing process, and that *Humana Conditio*, where he questions the motives of war, have become references for thinking about the concept of violence from his perspective.

On 8 May 1985, Norbert Elias was invited to give a lecture to commemorate the fortieth anniversary of the end of World War II by the University of Bielefeld, where he had been a regular visitor since 1971, where he lived and worked as a permanent scholarship holder at the no Centro de Pesquisa Interdisciplinar [*Zentrum für interdisziplinäre Forschung*], between 1978 and 1984, and from where he received the title of doctor *Honoris Causa*. Just as the physicist Albert Einstein had asked Freud a few years before the outbreak of that war, Norbert Elias also addressed the motives of war. His lecture, published as a book *Humana Condition*, and Freud's answer to Einstein, published under the title *Why War?* [*Warung Krieg?*], are two texts that consider violence not only at the level of the individual but also in processes that occur in social and international relations. Their starting point is the existence of psychic mechanisms that serve as devices that coerce urges, and they virtually reach the same conclusion, namely that there is no international monopoly of the violence that directs pacification processes in the event of war between nation-states.

Between July and September 1932, at the invitation of the League of Nations and its Instituto of Intellectual Co-operation, Einstein and Freud exchanged correspondence with the aim of addressing the following question: "Is there any way of delivering mankind from the menace of war?" (Einstein *apud* Freud 1933: 199). In a context in which Europe was suffering the political and economic setbacks of World War I and the strong threat of the rise to power of the National Socialist Party – remembering that the parliament was set fire to on the night of 27 February 1933 and that on 5 March of that same year Hitler was elected chancellor – , Einstein proposed to answer a number of questions: "How is it these devices succeed so well in rousing men to such enthusiasm, even to sacrifice their lives?" (Einstein *apud* Freud 1933: 201) and "Is it possible to controle man's mental evolution as to make him proof against the psychoses of hate and destructiveness?" (Einstein *apud* Freud 1933: 201).

In response to the first question, Einstein sketches some answers. As for the other two, he leaves it up to Freud to try to answer them in the light of ideas from psychoanalysis, without failing to underline the existence of aggressive impulses and desires for hatred and destruction inherent in human beings. Einstein considered important the existence of an institution that supported by an international agreement, played a legislative and legal role in conflicts between nations:

> the setting up, by international consent, of a legislative and judicial body to settle every conflict arising between nations. Each nation would undertake to abide by the orders issued by this legislative body, to invoke its decision in every dispute, to accepts its judgements unreservedly and to carry out every measure the tribunal deems necessary for the execution of its decrees.
>
> (Einstein *apud* Freud 1933: 199–200)

In this case it would be necessary for nations, as well as individuals, to abdicate part of their freedom and sovereignty, attributing the monopoly of violence to a supranational institution.

In reply to Einstein's letter, Freud talks about war and the ways of managing conflicts, as well as bout the psychic violence that individuals inflict on each other. If the German physicist proposes a discussion about law and power, Freud immediately replaces the word "power" with "violence" since, for him, power emerges as the development of violence. A path that has led from the free exercise of physical force towards its coercion via the law: "Violence could be broken by union, and the power of those who were united now represented law in contrast to the violence of the single individual. Thus we see that right is the might of a community" (Freud 1933: 205), Freud states. Power and violence, therefore, are not opposing terms.

Violence is neutralized by the appropriation of weapons that serve to intimidate and coerce. Later, it is replaced by the law and by justice, the power of a community. Violence against individuals is symbolically transformed into law as it becomes a way of states protecting individuals from the use of physical force against each other. Every individual must renounce power and transfer it to the state. "Wars will only be prevented with certainty if mankind unites in setting up a central authority to which the right of giving judgment upon all conflicts of interest shall be handed over" (Freud 1933: 207). By forming social organizations, individuals feel protected from the violence the emerges in human relationships. However, communities are formed via different power relations, with the result that the law also ends up being the exercise of this social inequality. Laws are made by those who dominate, and have little concern for the dominated, Freud concludes.

Sigmund Freud offers an extension of Weberian theses, just as Norbert Elias does, relating to the monopolization of violence by the state and the pacification of society. Consequently, in a proposition that we could call the *psychoanalytical theory of the civilizing process*, Freud sees civilization as a process that tends to control or at least reduce the effects of destruction impulses.

> The psychical modifications that go along with the process of civilization are striking and unambiguous. They consist in a progressive displacement of instinctual aims and a restriction of instinctual impulses. Sensations which were pleasurable to our ancestors have become indifferent or even intolerable to ourselves; there are organic grounds for the changes in our ethical and aesthetic ideals. Of the psychological characteristics of civilization two appear to be the most important: a strengthening of the intellect, which is beginning to govern instinctual life, and an internalization of the aggressive impulses, with all its consequent advantages and perils.
>
> (Freud 1933: 215)

The use of coercive force by an authority ensures the continued unity of a community of people driven by narcissisms and the drives to hate and destroy that are impossible to eliminate and can only be diverted and mitigated. In turn, to avoid war between states, it should also be their duty to renounce their individual powers in favour of a higher institution. The latter, he argues, holds the monopoly on legitimate use of power and force, inhibiting states from using violence against each other to further particular interests of sovereignty.

> The League of Nations is designed as an agency of this kind, but the second condition has not been fulfilled: the League of Nations has no power of its own and can only acquire it if the members of the new union, the separate states, are ready to resign it. And at the moment there seems very little prospect of this.
>
> (Freud 1933: 208)

Albert Einstein and Sigmund Freud, through the letters they exchanged, as well as Norbert Elias, in *Humana Conditio*, appear to agree that, to avoid war, the monopoly of violence, and the control of urges that lead states to create violent conflicts between each other falls to a higher entity. In the case of states, this power is exercised over individuals, even though within a community the solution to violence has never been avoided. As regards the relationship between states, no institution has been able to take on the same role.

In his lecture, published as the book *Humana Conditio*, Elias returns to the subject of violence, arguing that the self-control mechanisms that govern urges, developed throughout the civilizing process, have not been able to eliminate violent conflicts between human beings. Consequently "Wars are part of a fixed tradition of humanity. They are anchored in its social institutions and in the social habitus, the we-image, of people – even the most peace-loving people" (Elias 1985: 78). As a result of the threat that human beings represent to each other when they put in danger the place of hegemony and power, wars end up being caused by pressure from social institutions and by the formation of certain *habitus*. Added to this are the collective fantasies of greatness and superiority that inflate individuals' narcissistic emotions and end up creating social myths: "It is, of course, frightening that a cruel and pitiless social myth, provided it flattered the national pride of a people and satisfied a nation's need for confirmation of its unique value, could appeal to so many" (Elias 1985: 90). In the name of national myths, that preach an ideology of supremacy and bathe the members of a state in a *furor hegemonialis*, men have waged the bloodiest wars.

Spurred on by this hegemonic intoxication, as Elias called it, states are not content if they do not have the guarantee that their superiority is not under threat. Collective fantasies ultimately feed the ideal that both the state and individuals are destined for greatness via the domination of all others, whether via divine order or history or violence. Through the formation of social *habitus*, the ideals of the group, the state or the nation to which they belong are passed on to individuals:

> It is the case that all individuals carry with them in their personal habitus peculiarities of the habitus of their group, and that the fate of each individual person is partly determined by the fate and the reputation of groups to which he or she belongs.
>
> (Elias 1985: 108).

The search and the maintenance of the ideal of autonomy and sovereignty have found in the age-old tradition of resolving conflicts via the use of physical force, a way of eliminating neighbouring states and reducing their hegemonic powers. Militarization and the potential of armaments have become elements that have contributed to modern states forming a national image that is proud of itself, passing on to their individuals the idea that, as a consequence, they are secure and can consider themselves superior and better than the others.

If at an inter-state level states wish to monopolize violence, it cannot be said that the same is possible at an international level. Among themselves, states are always prepared for the use of physical violence in life-or-death struggles, destroying and killing their enemies whenever they feel threatened.

Until now, no international institution has been able to assume the monopoly of violence to guarantee pacification. Modern states received the traditions that constituted them as absolutist states governed by princes and kings who held the power to decide between war and peace. At the time when monarchic states were replaced by nation-states, the principles that all states must uphold their autonomy and sovereignty was passed on to the new governors. States are always ready for conflict since each of them represents a constant danger of becoming more powerful and stronger than the other. Therefore, in *Humana Conditio*, one of the conclusions that Norbert Elias reaches, repeated throughout this text from the very start, is that war is not a historical accident, but is part of the human condition: "the violent disputes between people, which we call wars, have been a part of the fate of human beings, of their conditions of life, for as far back as we can see. Human-made sorrow, human-made horror" (Elias 1985: 78). War is a human condition, subject to pressures from institutions and *social habitus*, part of the relationships between human beings and will probably be destined to continue to occur inevitably.

5.2 The times of trauma

It was during the period of World War I that Freud's thinking began to experience one if its most significant shifts. It was then that, with a great deal of time on his hands to speculate, he devoted himself almost entirely to writing. In October 1914 he began work on his well-known case "The Wolf Man", about a patient of his between 1910 and 1914, which was only published in 1918. Between March and May 1915, he wrote seven meta-psychological essays of which only five were published. In this same period the text *Thoughts for the Times on War and Death* (Freud 1915) also appeared. Between October and March 1915–1916 and 1916–1917, Freud also taught some courses on psychoanalysis at the Faculty of Medicine at the University of Vienna. In total 28 of his classes were published as the first *Introductory Lectures on Psychoanalysis*.

In 1918, with the decrease in battles, especially on the Eastern front, the entry into the war of the United States and the exit of Russia, the war appeared to be coming to an end. The Congresses of the IPA, which had been taking place since 1908, but which had to be suspended from 1913, were possible again. Life was gradually beginning to return to normal. Following much arguing over the location, it was decided that the Fifth International Psychoanalytic Congress would be held in Budapest between 28 and 29 September 1918. The effects of the death and destruction caused by the Great War had already begun to interest psychanalysts and psychoanalytic institutions. A few years earlier, in one of the introductory lectures, Freud announced to his audience:

> And now turn your eyes away from individuals and consider the Great War which is still laying Europe waste. Think of the vast amount of brutality, cruelty and lies which are able to spread over the civilized world. Do you really believe that a handful of ambitious and deluding men without conscience could have succeeded in unleashing all these evil spirits if their millions of followers did not share their guilt? Do you venture, in such circumstances, to break a lance on behalf of the exclusion of evil from the mental constitution of mankind?
>
> (Freud 1916–1917a: 146)

Given a call like this, the Fifth Congress focused on the theme of the *psychoanalysis of war neuroses*. Forty-two psychoanalysts took part, as well as members of the Austrian, German and Hungarian governments, who were interested in the subject in relation to military objectives. Sigmund Freud, Sándor Ferenczi, Karl Abraham, and Ernst Simmel were the speakers. Freud, in the lecture he gave at the congress, published under the title *Lines of Advance in Psycho-analytic Therapy*

(Freud 1919), stated that the day would come when society would recognise that the poor have as much right to psychological support and that psychic suffering affects the health of society as much as any other disease.

Consequently, aspects of the population's mental health, so-called war neuroses, became the main issue for discussion at that moment in time. In the introduction that he wrote for the publication that collated the papers delivered at the Fifth International Psychoanalytic Congress, Freud presented this new psychic category, seeking to consider it in relation to so-called common neuroses and traumatic neuroses that occurred in peace time. To do so he followed two lines of thought. For the first he stated that the ego is conflicted due to the schism between the "peaceful ego" and the "warlike ego" experienced especially by the average, totally unprepared citizen, when he is called up to go to war. Throughout their entire lives individuals have been led and coerced by social rules and by the state itself not to use physical violence, but in war time they are now obliged to kill their peers without mercy. Therefore, mostly against their will, they become transgressors of values that have defined their human condition, beyond barbarism, and have enabled them to create peaceful bonds in society.

> The conflict is between the soldier's old peaceful ego and his new warlike one, and it becomes acute as soon as the peace-ego realizes what danger it runs of losing its life owing to the rashness of its newly formed, parasitic double. It would be equally true to say that the old ego is protecting itself from a mortal danger by taking flight into a traumatic neurosis or to say that it is defending itself against the new ego which it sees is threatening its life. Thus the precondition of the war neuroses, the soil that nourishes them, would seem to be a national [conscript] army; there would be no possibility of their arising in an army of professional soldiers or mercenaries.
>
> (Freud 1919: 209)

Freud's second line of thinking about the emergence of war neuroses is not linked to conflicts of the ego. "Apart from this, the war neuroses are only traumatic neuroses, which, as we know, occur in peacetime too after frightening experiences or severe accidents, without any reference to a conflict in the ego" (Freud 1919: 209). Based on war neuroses, the idea of trauma, that served Freud in his development of the first aetiology of psychoneuroses, is taken up again as a guiding concept for psychoanalysis. In traumatic situations, what we see are symptoms caused by accidents, mechanical shocks, disasters, wartime events, etc. Any kind of event that delivers a blow that is impossible for the psyche to defend itself against in advance or to deal with. By being absorbed with the intensity and shock of the event, the defenceless, unprotected ego turns to sickness, normally physical, as a form of protection. Traumatic symptoms thus become attempts to give meaning, to represent something that, given its magnitude, could not be understood by the psyche.

Based on the formulations about narcissism and returning to the concept of trauma, war neuroses are considered narcissist disturbances that have made the ego sick as it has found itself in a position of vulnerability and unprepared. The ego recognizes the intensity of the shock as something dangerous and threatening, causing a neurosis that does not relate to ego conflict or defence mechanisms.

> In traumatic and war neuroses the human ego is defending itself from a danger which threatens it from without or which is embodied in a shape assumed by the ego itself. In the transference neuroses of peace the enemy from which the ego is defending itself is actually the libido, whose demands seem to it to be menacing. In both cases the ego is afraid of being damaged-in the latter case by the libido and in the former by external violence.
>
> (Freud 1919: 210)

Traumatic neuroses that can occur in war time or peace time, are instances of psychic suffering that seek to resolve in the body a conflict that, due to its violent nature, was incapable of leading to any kind of psychic representation. In the case of trauma, together with the lack of preparedness and vulnerability of the ego, the intensity, force, and instantaneous nature of the shock mark a reality that affects the ego as something irreducible. The traumatic event therefore turns into an "external" one that remains "within", like a foreign body that resists being metabolized or expelled by the organism. As Freud had already declared in one of his *Introductory Lectures*,

> The closest analogy to this behaviour of our neurotics is afforded by illnesses which are being produced with special frequency precisely at the present time by the war-what are described as traumatic neuroses. Similar cases, of course, appeared before the war as well, after railway collisions and other alarming accidents involving fatal risks. Traumatic neuroses are not in their essence the same thing as the spontaneous neuroses which we are in the habit of investigating and treating by analysis; nor have we yet succeeded in bringing them into harmony with our views, and I hope I shall be able at some time to explain to you the reason for this limitation. But in one respect we may insist that there is a complete agreement between them. The traumatic neuroses give a clear indication that a fixation to the moment of the traumatic accident lies at their root... It is as though these patients had not finished with the traumatic situation, as though they were still faced by it as an immediate task which has not been dealt with; and we take this view quite seriously. It shows us the way to what we may call an economic view of mental processes. Indeed, the term 'traumatic' has no other sense than an economic one. We apply it to an experience which within a short period of time presents the mind with an increase of stimulus too powerful to be dealt with or worked off in the normal way, and this must result in permanent disturbances of the manner in which the energy operates.
>
> (Freud 1916–191b: 274–275)

It will take another few years, as well as a lot of courage for Freud to solve the problem that, in this paper, he could not resolve for his audience. A step forward was taken in returning to something that was the basis of his thinking right at the beginning of his first theories about psychoanalytical practice. The return to traumatic causality in the formation of psychic symptoms, fundamental for the early days of psychoanalysis between 1895 and 1897, and a new understanding of the economy of the psychic apparatus are key to developing an understanding about what could lead to people becoming sick who have been through extremely violent experiences. Consequently, in his text *Beyond the Pleasure Principle* [*Jenseits des Lustprinzips*], of 1920, based on the account of traumatic dreams and symptoms presented in his sessions with former combatants from World War I, psychoanalytical theory reached a new level in terms of the relationship between individuals and society, consolidating the concept of trauma as acting to suspend any division between the interior and the exterior, the internal, and the external worlds, the ego and the other, body, and psyche. However, it is no longer a question of considering trauma as the product of a violent act of a sexual nature, by an adult individual on a seduced child, nor of tracing trauma back to shock theory, as 19th century psychiatry had done, as Freud states:

> A condition has long been known and described which occurs after severe mechanical concussions, railway disasters and other accidents involving a risk to life; it has been given the name of l "traumatic neurosis". The terrible war which has just ended gave rise to a great number of illnesses of this kind, but it at least put an end to the temptation to attribute the cause of the disorder to organic lesions of the nervous system brought about by mechanical force.
>
> (Freud 1920: 12)

Supported by a new theory of drives, now divided between the life drive [*Lebenstrieb*] and the death drive [*Todestrieb*], the understanding of trauma as the external impact of violent intensity on a psychic system returns definitively to revise the entire economic theory of metapsychology put forward up to that point. In the case of traumatic neuroses, Freud emphasizes a factor that has a decisive influence on the production of this structure. Fright or terror [*Schreck*], as an unexpected factor, catches the individual unprepared to deal with or defend themselves against a violent experience or one with a high emotional charge.

Due to the lack of preparedness to deal with an extremely strong stimulus, one that is so powerful that it ruptures protective structures and does not permit any kind of elaboration, the psychic apparatus remains unable to establish any kind of connection with or new representations of the traumatic experience. "We may, I think, tentatively venture to regard the common traumatic neurosis as a consequence of an extensive breach being made in the protective shield against stimuli" (Freud 1920: 31), Freud states. The violence directly attacks the protective structure of the psyche. The traumatic shock represents the failure of the ego's control and defence mechanisms. It makes the psyche work on forming traumatic symptoms as a way of reorganizing the undermined psychic economy. In the words of Freud,

> We describe as "traumatic" any excitations from outside which are powerful enough to break through the protective shield, It seems to me that the concept of trauma necessarily implies a connection of this kind with a breach in an otherwise efficacious barrier against stimuli. Such an event as an ex ternal trauma is bound to provoke a disturbance on a large scale in the functioning of the organism's energy and to set in motion every possible defensive measure. At the same time, the pleasure principle is for the moment put out of action. There is no longer any possibility of preventing the mental apparatus from being flooded with large amounts of stimulus, and another problem arises instead the problem of mastering the amounts. of stimulus which have broken in and of binding them, in the psychical sense, so that they can then be disposed of.
>
> (Freud 1920: 29–30)

We therefore return to the point that we have just described: external stimuli are so powerful that they rupture any protection of the psychic apparatus; they become traumatic, as the functioning of the psychic economy is diminished; however, the pleasure principle does not function as it normally does with the other psychic structures; and, instead of the attacked ego, incapable of offering any kind of connection with or representation of the traumatic event, the psychic apparatus has to find another way of eliminating the amount of energy that suddenly materialises.

By analyzing the dreams of former war combatants, but also children's play and anxiety dreams, Freud was able to recognize that the pleasure principle was not the main mechanism for resolving psychic conflicts. Neither was it the pleasure principle that led the individual to return to the scene of the trauma, since the trauma in fact never produced any sensation of pleasure. According to Freud, repetition compulsion [*Wiederholungszwang*] leads to traumatic symptoms to fulfil other purposes:

> But it is impossible to classify as wish-fulfilments the dreams we have been discussing which occur in traumatic neuroses, or the dreams during psychoanalyses which bring to memory the psychical traumas of childhood. They arise, rather, in obedience to the compulsion to repeat, though it is true that in analysis that compulsion is supported by the wish (which is encouraged by 'suggestion') to conjure up what has been forgotten and repressed.
>
> (Freud 1920: 32)

According to this new change in Freudian economy theory, the psychic apparatus was no longer solely at the service of the pleasure principle. It also acts as a force for preservation which tends to repetition. "the patient is, one might say, fixated to his trauma" (Freud 1920: 13), Freud writes. Re-living the traumatic scene is to repeat it and process and elaborate infinitely to prevent the collapse of the psychic system in the face of the excessive emotional charge caused during the trauma. Fractures, ruptures and disconnections return bringing back into the present situations of pain, suffering and death. Freud therefore concluded that the death drive leads to repetitions of the traumatic scene to elaborate the unbearable nature of a reality within a possible reality.

Shortly after, in *Inhibition, Symptom and Anxiety*, new elaborations were put forward about trauma. What was considered the result of a traumatic situation caused by the ego's lack of preparedness in situations of extreme violence was ultimately understood as a primordial feature of human beings. The ego's fragility and the limits of its dependence on other individuals, from birth onwards, leaves it in a state of helplessness [*Hilflosigkeit*] in the face of dangers with external or internal origins, dangers whose excesses of emotional charges can come to manifest themselves as traumatic situations. Anxiety, in turn, becomes a device that the ego uses to announce the occurrence of this danger and thus prepare to protect itself from the repetition of the same traumatic event previously experienced. Freud explains as follows:

> Taking this sequence, anxiety-danger-helplessness (trauma), we can now summarize what has been said. A danger-situation is a recognized, remembered, expected situation of helplessness. Anxiety is the original reaction to helplessness in the trauma and is reproduced later on in the danger situation as a signal for help. The ego, which experienced the trauma passively, now repeats it actively in a weakened version, in the hope of being able itself to direct its course... After that come the later displacements, from the danger to the determinant of the danger-loss of the object and the modifications of that loss with which we are already acquainted.
>
> (Freud 1926: 166–167)

The ego's state of helplessness becomes the foundation of the traumatic situation, unprotected to deal with any dangerous situation that unexpectedly crops up. At that point Freud tries to attenuate the difference between traumatic neuroses and those of transference, showing that the totality of the ego is always threatened, whether in a situation of external danger, as in war time, where there is a very real possibility of actual death, or whether in a situation of internal danger, where the ego feels threatened with the possibility of disappearing in a subjective death. When the origin of the danger comes from within, what is at issue is the separation or the loss of the ego of a loved one who gave it protection. There are various events that during an individual's life align with the loss of a protective object and thus precipitating traumatic situations throughout life: birth, separation from the mother, the fear of losing the caregiver's love, the fear of losing the love of the superego.

Throughout the development of the ego, this loss shifts from the *fear of the loss of the other* to the *fear of the loss of their love* and, subsequently, to *social fear*, when the individual feels threatened with losing the protection of the group that they form part of. In this sense, trauma presents itself as a situation in which all individuals experience, in one way or another, the separation from someone who has provided care, protection, and support. The important point to underline, in this theoretical aspect, is that situations of social violence, that cause psychic helplessness, may evoke unconscious memories of individual traumatic experiences in which the ego found itself in a position of fragility and lacking protection. The boundaries between the social and the psychic, between the subjective and the political, and between the individual and society end up being suspended.

Despite Freudian theory about trauma undergoing many modifications in the course of his work, the idea that trauma always inscribes itself via a dual temporality is unequivocal. Freud's reading of trauma did not only disrupt the borders between the social and the psychic, the clinical and the political, the self and the other, the individual and society, but also presented a new temporality in the order of signification of events, which is neither absolute rupture with the past nor one of linear progression. In his first reflections on the formation of psychic trauma as the cause of neurotic symptoms, in the late 1890s, Freud identified in the accounts given by his patients the existence of a first moment in time when a violent act, mostly of a sexual nature and caused by real agents, impacted on the child by inflicting a certain amount of excitement that they could not yet understand. An act of sexual violence caused by an authoritarian other affected an objectified, weakened body that was still incapable of giving any kind of meaning to the act.

This "foreign body" whose excess of energy invaded the childlike a powerful shock, however, only becomes traumatizing element at a second, subsequent moment in time. The time of trauma is the time of *deferred action* [*Nachträglichkeit*], which is produced by the repetition of this event as an act in the present time or as a memory of a past event. Events that have been repressed, Freud argues, are neither destroyed nor eradicated. They are preserved in the unconscious, from where they can produce symptoms and repetitions. The past event remains preserved and active in the present time as a traumatic situation. In this second time when it is remembered, the time of *a posteriori*, a scene recalls a memory, re-signifying the original event as an act of violence. It can, therefore, be said that Freudian theory about trauma also breaks with the linearity of time and causality, as the past ceases to be an event independent from the present by being brought back into the present when it is re-signified.

For Norbert Elias, the notions of past, present, and future cannot be defined as a sequence of events integrated into a regular, uniform, and continuous flow, or as separate, self-contained, temporal representations, as they are imbricated in *lived experience*. A more in-depth study of the way he understands our relationship with time can be found in the text *Time: an essay* [*Über die Zeit*]. According to this text, the constant course of change in our lived experiences inscribes a future of significations in which no moment is obviously determined. Elias writes: "What is past merges seamlessly with the present, as the present does with the future. This is seen clearly enough when the future, having become the present, becomes in its turn the past" (Elias 1984: 81). Past, present, and future, through being intrinsically linked to the human experience, ultimately constitute the same, single concept, Elias concludes.

In some passages of *The Germans*, we see chronological linearity being distanced from lived experiences, for example when Elias refers to the past as an event that is updated like an "echo" (Elias 1989: 346) in the present; or when he states that "the past also throws a shadow over political deeds and thoughts" (Elias 1989: 260); or when he emphasises the force of the past on the present:

> The pattern of its past, its chances and expectations for the future play just as great a role as determinants of a nation's conduct here and now as does the immediate present. In this as in other respects, the past leaves its imprint on the present order and ways of behaving. It does so implicitly as one of their conditions, explicitly through the image which living generations carry with them of their country's past. As determinants of behaviour, past, present and future work together. Lived situations, as it were, are three-dimensional.
>
> (Elias 1989: 355)

In the following excerpt, Elias appears to illustrate the suspension of the linear, progressive, and divided temporality of lived experiences:

> But the past is never simply the past. It works on – with greater or lesser force according to circumstances – as an influence in the present. It does so not only because of the inertia of traditions which roll blindly on, but also because an image of past phases of one's own society, distorted and deformed though it may be, continues to live on in the consciousness of subsequent generations, serving involuntarily as a mirror in which one can see oneself.
>
> (Elias 1989: 53)

In Elias's view, past societies remain active in present-day societies via social institutions, which are preserved and passed on in the form of habits, behaviours, and thoughts which, in most cases, we do not know the origins or intentions of.

The past seems to never cease to present itself as current, actively making itself present, whether via the formation of psychic symptoms or social habits, for example. The effects of histories that have helped shape nation-states, notably the histories of wars and conquests, victories and defeats, expansions and ruptures, dominations and submission, are passed on to shape the personality of their members. Therefore, in his research Norbert Elias describes a series of situations that marked the life of a nation at the same time as determining the drive economy and the self-control mechanisms of its citizens. Memories that were recorded as vestiges in the history of the individual and in the history of society, imposing the need to be revisited whenever they are silenced, forgotten, and repressed due to their traumatic or violent aspects. A social trauma thus becomes a psychic one.

This brings us back to times of war and violence to think about the effects of the rupturing of the link between state and individual. Wars destroy, with a single blow, all civilizing pacts: "We cannot but feel that no event has ever destroyed so much that is precious in the common possessions of humanity, confused so many of the clearest intelligences, or so thoroughly debased what is highest" (Freud 1915: 275). In Freud's view, states at war above all wish to take possession of individuals' relative freedom to force them to serve their own interests of sovereignty by threatening death and exclusion. All they do is destroy the guarantees that individuals have of recognizing themselves as people and as citizens.

> A belligerent state permits itself every such misdeed, every such act of violence, as would disgrace the individual. It makes use against the enemy not only of the accepted *ruses de guerre*, but of deliberate lying and deception as well – and to a degree which seems to exceed the usage of former wars. The state exacts the utmost degree of obedience and sacrifice from its citizens, but at the same time it treats them like children by an excess of secrecy and a censorship upon news and expressions of opinion which leaves the spirits of those whose intellects it thus suppresses defenceless against every unfavourable turn of events and every sinister rumour. It absolves itself from the guarantees and treaties by which it was bound to other states, and confesses shamelessly to its own rapacity and lust for power, which the private individual has then to sanction in the name of patriotism.
>
> (Freud 1915: 279)

Given this, whether in peace time or war time, states position themselves as agents that produce traumatic situations when they are unable to exercise the monopolies that they have become responsible to. Allowing social exclusions, economic privileges and political perversities to occur, the state itself produces situations of violence, in most cases against those individuals who do not represent the hegemonic features of the established group that holds the power. Instead of protecting its members and providing social equality, the state becomes a perpetrator and inciter of violence, dismantling all forms of regulation of urges that have been constructed throughout the civilizing process. In the name of its sovereignty, the state breaks with the truth and with the exercise of notions like solidarity, civility, and respect for life, authorizing and forming a pact with the use of cruel, barbaric, and inhuman behaviour. The violence of states obliges human beings to reveal the most hostile and aggressive aspects of their nature, reducing citizens to instruments for serving its own interests.

5.3 The two sides of the coin: civilization and decivilization

Elias's theory of civilizing processes was first formulated "precisely at the time when Hitler was refuting the argument on the grandest scale" (Leach 1986). As Stephen Mennell (2001) reminds us, with this statement the British anthropologist Sir Edmund Leach tried to discredit one of the most important sociological works of the 20th century. His critique was based on the fact that *The Civilizing Process* had been published in the same year as Nazi Germany invaded Poland, without making any references to the retrograde developments that were then already pointing to the greatest atrocities that humanity would go on to witness. In fact, Norbert Elias, along with many other thinkers, did not foresee the barbarism that was about to take place.

In 1935, before definitively going into exile, Elias was in his home country for the last time. At that point, as he himself recalled, the swastika symbol was increasingly seen dotted around the city. However, even with the arrival of the National Socialist Party in power, says Elias, "Conditions in Germany were still well ordered, and the feeling that it was a constitutional state where no harm could come to you was deeply rooted" (Elias 1990: 51). Elias's parents, for example, refused his invitation to stay with him in England, preferring to return to their home in Germany. They still had friends in Breslau, a life to be lived, and they thought that, as they had never harmed anyone, nothing could happen to them. As we know, the last time that Elias met his parents in person was in 1938 when they went to visit him in England. His father Hermann Elias died from ill-health in 1940, and his mother Sophie Elias was taken to a concentration camp, where she was executed in a gas chamber.

Norbert Elias did attend a Hitler rally in Frankfurt, between the end of 1932 and the beginning of 1933. This experience had a considerable impact on him in terms of coming face to face with alterity. The arrival of the *Führer* was marked with patriotic songs by the mass of adoring supporters, as Elias himself recalled (Elias 1987: 45). He felt obliged to move his lips to avoid looking like the only one remaining silent. Disguised by a hunter's hat so that his nose looked less Jewish, looking like a tramp and accompanied by two other students, he managed to get through the SS barrier to await the Nazi leader, who fascinated the German people. Hitler represented the leader who could rouse people with his speeches, making Germany a united country again after successive defeats in wars and conflicts.

Nevertheless, his exile in England, his work at the London School of Economics and his transfer to Cambridge made Elias's life a little more comfortable. "There we led the most peaceful of lives, punting on the river, and drinking coffee and tea in a nearby village. It was a thoroughly peaceful 'phoney war'". (Elias 1990: 62). If this statement, as David Rotman said, resulted from the "it is certainly also the distorting effect of a retrospective illusion" (2005: 151), the fact is that Elias was becoming an outsider again, living in a country whose immigration control policy was increasingly suspicious of the refugees it was playing host to. In 1939, when England officially declared war on Germany, almost 70,000 Austrian and German citizens immediately had their visas revoked and were declared *enemy aliens*. The same happened to around 8,000 Italian exiles, after war was declared in Italy in 1940. They were all immediately transferred to internment camps dotted all over England. Norbert Elias was taken to a camp located on the Isle of Man, where he was held for almost six months, between May and October 1940. Due to his Jewish origins, Elias was obliged to leave his country to save himself from Nazi persecution. Due to his German nationality, he was again considered an enemy and detained alongside many other foreigners. A dual status of outsider meant that he was a pariah in the eyes of the nation that hosted him and in those of his nation of origin, that persecuted him.

Undoubtedly life in British internment camps bore absolutely no relation to what was going on in German concentration camps, namely forced labour and the extermination of the Jewish people, as well as many other groups. In England the camps were housed in civic buildings, like hotels and guest houses, and the occupants themselves carried out the administrative duties, organizing the domestic chores necessary for community life. As a way of resisting a life of restrictions and confinement, the interned organized teaching and learning activities where they could use and pass on their diverse knowledge: agriculture and economics, as well as languages and general knowledge, like history, the humanities, law, mathematics, and theology. Norbert Elias, for example, taught art history, social psychology, psychoanalysis, and sociology. A musical comedy entitled *What a life!* narrating scenes from daily life, was organized and performed by those interned in one of the camps.

Even so, the principles of a concentration camp still applied. Persecution, the removal of personal objects and autonomy, limits on free time and movement within the physical space, privations in terms of food and contact with others, the withdrawal of individual identities in favour of treating all prisoners as a mass, and control of social and sexual pleasure were all elements that brought the English internment camps in line with totalitarian institutions. The deconstruction of self-image, together with a dual severing of identifications caused by Nazi persecution of Jews and German citizens led to severe psychic suffering, which in many cases ended in suicide.

Edmund Leach seems not to have understood the meaning of the concept of the civilizing process presented in the *magnum opus* of figurational theory, going as far as to state that this theory was, in his view, very Germanic and shaped by ideas about a long-term social process which dated from the 19th century. Elias did not fail to consider the darkness of that time, as can be seen in the preface to *The Civilizing Process*, written in 1936:

> However, the issues raised by the book have their origin less in scholarly tradition, in the narrower sense of the word, than in the experiences in whose shadow we all live, experiences of the crisis and transformation of Western civilization as it had existed hitherto, and the simple need to understand what this "civilization" really amounts to.
>
> (Elias 1939: xiv)

According to Elias, civilizing processes take place in a blind, unforeseen way, always permeated by retrograde movements caused by decivilizing impulses. It is only possible to understand them as an interplay of contradictory forces in which, sometimes, at a given point in history, one prevails over the other. What Leach stated about figurational theory presupposes that Elias was incapable of considering movements contrary to the formation of civilizing ties, especially those that reach the level of barbarism. Leach, however, seems not to have taken into account the fact that Elias was always alert to the insecurities and violent acts that are part of the daily life of individuals and of relationships between states.

As Jonathan Fletcher (1997) describes, the civilizing process follows three paths: a change in the balance between the restrictions imposed by others and self-restraint involving domestication; differentiation and the increase in complexity of external controls; the development of a social standard of behaviour and sentiment that generates the emergence of a more uniform, encompassing, stable, and differentiated self-coercion; an increase in the reach of mutual identification between people. However, insecurity, lack of protection and fear are conditions that, even in highly peaceful societies, never disappear. They are not eliminated by the civilizing process, but rather transferred to the background of individuals' psychic lives and of the public life of societies.

Jonathan Fletcher (1997: 85) also suggests some criteria, logically implicit in the theory of civilizing processes, to describe decivilizing processes: a shift in the balance between the restrictions of others and self-restraint in favour of the restrictions of others; the development of a social standard of behaviour and sentiment that generates the emergence of a more uniform, encompassing, stable, and differentiated level of self-restraint; and a contraction in the scope of mutual identification between constituent groups and individuals. Decivilizing processes normally come to prominence in conditions in which there is a reduction in state control of violence, when there is fragmentation of social ties, and a shortening of the chain of interdependence between people. In these cases, fear, lack of protection and insecurity, the increase in violence and aggression in the public sphere, the increase in inequalities, and in the power imbalances between different social classes end up being some of the effects of the decivilizing process.

After analyzing the civilizing process of France and England, the conceptual basis of the relationship between established and outsider groups, during the first half of the 1960s, was fundamental for investigating the formation of the German State. Thus, in *The Germans*, Elias's last great work published in his lifetime, topics like intolerance and social exclusion were present in the formation of the structures of the society and the personality of the German people, and the Jewish question, in turn, involved the author of the work himself in a life marked by exclusions and acts of silencing.

When applying his theory about the established/outsiders configuration, the place of the Jew bears the mark of the excluded, of the foreigner, and of the hatred of the other. The problem of the German Jews was effectively a problem of relations between established and outsider groups. Like many other outsider groups, Jews were excluded in imperial Germany from a whole range of social promotions. Consequently, in *The Germans* we again find an analysis of the power relations between different social groups and the consequences caused by those who seek to maintain their privileges and power.

Jews have always occupied marginal spaces in European societies. However, according to accounts by Elias himself (1990), in the time of Wilhelm II, the last German emperor, belonging to that group did not appear to be a major problem. Despite the discrimination and stigmatization directed at Jews, a degree of physical, economic, and cultural security still gave them a certain guarantee of protection. In Breslau, Elias's father, who originated from a Prussian town where the majority of the population were Jews, worked as a businessman in the textile sector and was part of an autonomous class within the local bourgeoisie. Elias himself, in his youth, saw himself as a member both of the German community and of the Jewish community, without needing to establish many differences between the two groups. This was a perception that, in his words, represented self-blindness, an illusion of someone who experienced a world of safety without recognizing the real antisemitism that existed in the upper echelons of society: "The Jewish community must have been blind, but blinded partly because they were prosperous" (Elias 1990: 13). This world of total protection would only change for Elias with the advent of World War I, when the rupture of the civilizing pact sparked fear and insecurity that until then seemed to be unshakeable.

Stephen Mennell (1997) contends that Judaism was a fundamental driver of the research that Norbert Elias carried out throughout his trajectory, even if this idea was further applied to research on the relationship between class differences, racial and ethnic issues, power relations between men and women, and the most varied configurations that are established between individuals. Following this same line of thought, Nathalie Heinich (2014) states that the Jewish question was already present in Elias's own life well before it became a subject of his research, to the extent that it shaped his relationships when he was a young student who was mixing in student groups in Germany. In Heinich's view there is a silencing of the themes of Jew and Judaism in Elias's other works, that, in *The Germans*, end up being "It is the starting point, the invisible foundation of all his work", in other words, "its central problem – how to deal with inclusion and exclusion when you are Jewish – and the central problem of the man who produced it" (Heinich 2014: 290). For Heinich, however, the main theme of *The Germans*, and Elias's work as a whole, deals with the processes of inclusion and exclusion of individuals, or to put it another way, the psychic and social effects of individuals' moving from lower social classes to higher ones. She stresses that this process results in suffering and symptoms in social and psychic structures.

Elias, however, does not position the Jewish question and antisemitism at the centre of his analyses, nor does he situate Jews as a key element to understanding the retrograde evolution of civilization in Hitler's Germany. He is also conscious that other genocides occurred in the 20th century and that the Jews were not the only victims of this type of barbarism. The collection of texts brought together in *The Germans*, furthermore, does not simply amount to the investigation of the course of the formation of the German state, as if the transformations of the social structures could be separated from the changes in psychic structures. For Norbert Elias, analyses of societies must necessarily be accompanied by the examination of individuals' drive economy. In this way, at the same time as he describes the sociogenesis of Germany, he also focuses on the study of the psychogenesis of the German people.

In fact, on recovering historical and social elements that helped to shape that country's *national habitus*, Elias aims to answer the following question "what is it to be German?" – posed for the first time in the context of *The Civilizing Process*, and posed again in *The Germans* – in order to reflect on the decivilizing process that led to the formation of the Third Reich and the barbaric acts perpetrated by the Nazis. This research includes the violence of the drive demands in the political sphere, illustrating that social bonds transmit forms of love between those who are identical and expressions of hate between those who are different. Norbert Elias, therefore, proposes thinking that the civilizing process is accompanied by regressive movements caused by the decivilizing process, with the result that, between one and the other, there is a balance that sometimes swings more to one side and at other times more to the other.

References

Elias, Norbert (1939) *The Civilizing Process. Sociogenetic and Psychogenetic Investigations*, ed. by E. Dunning, J. Goudsblom and S. Mennell, trans. by E. Jephcott. Oxford: Blackwell Publishing, 2013.

——— (1984) *Time: An Essay*, trans. by E. Jephcott. Oxford/Cambridge: Blackwell, 1992.

——— (1984–85) "Sociology... Done in the Right Way", in *Collected Work of Norbert Elias: Interviews and Autobiographical Reflections*, ed. by E. Jephcott, R. Kilminster, K. Liston and S. Mennell, trans. by E. Jephcott. Dublin: University College Dublin Press, 2012.

——— (1985) "Humana Conditio", in *The Collected Work of Norbert Elias – The Loneliness of the Dying and Humana Conditio*, vol. 6, ed. by A. and B. Scott, trans. by E. Jephcott. Dublin: University College Dublin Press, 2010.

——— (1987) *J'ai suivi mon propre chemin: un parcours dans le siècle*. Paris: Sociales Editions, 2016.

——— (1989) *The Germans. Power Struggles and the Development of Habitus in the Nineteenth and Twentieth Centuries*, trans. by E. Dunning and S. Mennell. New York: Columbia University Press, 1996.

——— (1990) *Reflections on a Life*, trans. by E. Jephcott. Cambridge: Polity Press, 1994.

Fletcher, Jonathan (1997) *Violence and Civilization. An Introduction to the Work of Norbert Elias*. Cambridge: Polity Press, 2005.

Freud, Sigmund (1908) "'Civilized' Sexual Morality and Modern Nervous Illness", in *The Standard Edition of the Complete Psychological Works of Sigmund Freud – Jensen's 'Gradiva' and Other Works (1906–1908)*, vol. IX, ed. and trans. by J. Strachey. London: Hogarth Press, 1981.

——— (1915) "Thought on the Times of War and Death", in *The Standard Edition of the Complete Psychological Work of Sigmund Freud – On the History of Psycho-Analytic Movement, Papers on Metapsychology and Other Works (1914–1916)*, vol. XIV, ed. and trans. by J. Strachey. London: Hogarth Press, 1981.

——— (1916–1917a) "The Censorship of Dreams", in *The Standard Edition of the Complete Psychological Works of Sigmund Freud – Introductory Lectures on Psycho-analysis (Parts I and II)*, vol. XV, ed. and trans. by J. Strachey. London: Hogarth Press, 1981.

——— (1916–1917b) "Fixation to Traumas – The Unconscious", in *The Standard Edition of the Complete Psychological Works of Sigmund Freud – Introductory Lectures on Psycho-analysis (Part III)*, vol. XVI, ed. and trans. by J. Strachey. London: Hogarth Press, 1981.

——— (1919) "Introduction to *Psycho-analysis and the War Neurosis*", in *The Standard Edition of the Complete Psychological Works of Sigmund Freud – An Infantile Neurosis and other Works (1917–1919)*, vol. XVII, ed. and trans. by J. Strachey. London: Hogarth Press, 1981.

——— (1920) "Beyond the Pleasure Principle", in *The Standard Edition of the Psychoanalytical Works of Sigmund Freud – Beyond the Pleasure Principle, Group Psychology and Other Works (1920–1922)*, vol. XVIII, ed. and trans. by J. Strachey. London: Hogarth Press, 1981.

——— (1926) "Inhibition, Symptoms and Anxiety", in *The Standard Edition of the Complete Psychological Works of Sigmund Freud – An Autobiographical Study, Inhibition,*

Symptoms and Anxiety, The Question of Lay Analysis and Other Works (1925–1926), vol. XX, ed. and trans. by J. Strachey. London: Hogarth Press, 1981.

——— (1933) "Why War", in *The Standard Edition of the Complete Work of Sigmund Freud – New Introductory Lectures on Psycho-analysis and Other Works (1932–1936)*, vol. XXII, ed. and trans. by J. Strachey. London: Hogarth Press, 1981.

Freud, Sigmund and Abraham, Karl (2002) *The Complete Correspondence of Sigmund Freud and Karl Abraham (1907–1925)*, trans. by C. Schwarzacher. London: Karnac.

Freud, Sigmund and Andreas-Salomé, Lou (1972) *Sigmund Freud and Lou Andreas-Salomé Letters*, ed. by E. Pfeiffer, trans. by W. and E. Robson-Scott. New York: Harcourt Brace Jovanovich.

Freud, Sigmund and Ferenczi, Sándor (1996) *The Complete Correspondence of Sigmund Freud and Sándor Ferenczi (1914–1919)*, vol. 2, trans. by P. Hoffer. London: The Belkap Press of Harvard University Press.

Heinich, Nathalie (2014) "Sublimer le ressentiment. Elias et les cinq voies vers une autre sociologie", in *Revue du MAUSS*, vol. 2014/2, n.44. www.cairn.info/revue-du-mauss-2014-2-page-289.htm.

Lacroix, Bernard (1997) "Portrait sociologique de l'auteur", in *Norbert Elias, la politique et l'histoire*. Paris: Éditions de la Découverte.

Leach, Edmund (1986 Oct.) "Violence", in *London Review of Books*, vol. 8, n.18. www.lrb.co.uk/the-paper/v08/n18/edmund-leach/violence.

Mennell, Stephen (1997) *Norbert Elias: An Introduction*. Dublin: University College of Dublin, 2010.

——— (2001) "The Other Side of the Coin: Decivilizing Processes", in *Norbert Elias and Human Interdependencies*, ed. by T. Salumets. Montreal/Québec: McGill-Queen's University Press.

Rotman, David (2005) "Trajectoire intellectuelle et expérience du camp: Norbert Elias à l'Île de Man", in *Revue d'histoire Moderne & Contemporaine*, vol. 2005/2, n.52–2.

6 Beyond the civilizing process

Just as Freud showed that symptomatic repetition is the expression of the destinies of the drive in each individual, Norbert Elias described national habitus as the expression of the destinies of the drive in each nation. Transferred to behind the scenes of psychic and social life, the erasure of a memory values and establishes hegemonic discourses that allow or prohibit access to social positions of privilege and recognition for certain individuals or certain social classes. Only then, in a process of memory reconstruction, when individuals and nations are confronted with their own history and their own past, is it possible to break the symptomatic series of repetitions that causes discontent and transmits and perpetuates trauma, violence and suffering against oneself and against others. Norbert Elias states in his work *The Germans*:

> It is not yet common practice today to link the current social and national habitus of a nation to its so-called 'history', and especially to the state-formation process it has experienced. Many people seem to have the unspoken opinion that "What happened in the twelfth, fifteenth or eighteenth centuries is past – what has it got to do with me?" In reality, though, the contemporary problems of a group are crucially influenced by their earlier fortunes, by their beginningless development.
>
> (1989: 19)

Much more than an analysis of the Jewish people, the work *The Germans* sets out to be a biography of the German State, investigating the formation processes of the German *national habitus* in order, through them, to think about the conditions that led to the violence of the decivilizing processes during the Third Reich. In fact, Elias's studies about the Germans are dedicated to researching the *national habitus*, but they give special emphasis to their transformations, marked by ruptures and discontinuities caused by centuries and centuries of wars, by class conflicts between the militarized aristocracy and the humanist bourgeoisie and the belated unification of the German state. It is from the continuities and discontinuities

DOI: 10.4324/9781003378938-6

within the formation of the German State that Elias analyzes the social conditions that made it possible for a large part of society to implement decivilizing forces towards intolerance and the annihilation of the other, as happened in the Nazi genocide carried out during the Third Reich.

To speak of a *decivilizing spurt* implies considering movements of *force* and *regression* that simultaneously appear as the two sides of the same coin, or the right and wrong of civilizing forces. In his work *The Germans*, Elias mentions the idea of "rebarbarization" or "regression to barbarism" to describe the direction of the decivilizing process. Would the civilized societies of the 20th century be living in a time of regression of civilization? How could Germany, such a civilized country, have been able to persecute and eliminate almost an entire people in such a cruel and inhuman way never witnessed before? "The whole war was clearly a regression to barbarism", says Elias. However, he continues,

> Up till then, however, European wars had always been relatively limited regressions. Certain minimum rules of civilized conduct were generally still observed even in the treatment of prisoners of war. With a few exceptions, a kernel of self-esteem which prevents the senseless torturing of enemies and allows identification with one's enemy in the last instance as another human being, together with compassion for his suffering, did not entirely lapse.
>
> (Elias 1989: 309)

With the events of World War I, Sigmund Freud completely transformed his theory on the principles of mental functioning. From then on, the psychic economy was no longer solely at the service of the pleasure principle. There were also regressive forces which did not direct the drive economy towards the obtaining of satisfactions. They were forces at the service of destruction and annihilation. In opposition to the pleasure principle, then, it is not the displeasure, but the death drive. The pure expression of aggressiveness.

On the eve of World War II, in a letter he wrote to the physicist Albert Einstein, entitled *Why War?* Freud (1933) takes up again his theory of drives to think about the conditions that led humanity to reach certain states of barbarism. His attempt was never to reduce or simplify the explanations about the reasons of wars to the economic principles of the psychic apparatus. But among these, for Freud, it is undeniable to include destructive tendencies, the death drive and aggressiveness. In the face of this, then, what can be said about the regression to barbarism produced by Hitler's German state, where death was at the service of the total destruction of life? Could we think of the pure expression of a death drive, of the elimination of all human ties between individuals and societies?

The outbreaks of destruction during the Hitler period cannot be considered pathological deviations either by individuals or societies, since they are part of the civilizing process of the German national state. Thus, in the light of the theory of civilizing processes, Elias includes the breakdown of civilization [*Der Zusammenbruch der Zivilisation*] as a result of the weakening of self-control mechanisms and superego elements in the identification processes of individuals with national ideals, intensifying the degree of fear and insecurity and promoting the return of socially weakened instinctual forces.

"The fortunes of a nation become crystallized in institutions", states Elias, so that "the most different people of a society acquire the same characteristics, possess the same national habitus" (1989: 18). Here is the central purpose of his work *The Germans*: to understand how the destinies of a nation are established throughout the centuries in the formation of *national habitus*. Once again, Freud is recognized by Elias as an important interlocutor to resolve this problem: "Sociologists face a task here which distantly recalls the task which Freud tackled" (Elias 1989: 19). Elias therefore proceeds to explain his proposal to go beyond Freud's thinking:

> He [Freud] attempted to show the connection between the outcome of the conflict-ridden channelling of drives in a person's development and his or her resulting habitus. But there are also analogous connections between a people's long-term fortunes and experiences and their social habitus at any subsequent time. At this layer of the personality structure – let us for the time being call it the 'we-layer' – there are often complex symptoms of disturbance at work which are scarcely less in strength and in capacity to cause suffering than the individual neuroses. In both cases it is a matter of bringing back into consciousness, quite often in the face of strong resistance, things which have been forgotten. In the one as in the other, such an undertaking requires a certain self-distancing, and may, if successful, contribute to the loosening of rigid models of behaviour.
>
> (Elias 1989: 19)

Freud died on 23 September 1939, just days after Germany invaded Poland, starting World War II. In the last months of his life, he was persecuted by his nation, had his books burned in the public square, and was forced to leave the city where he had lived for most of his life. But Freud did not witness the greatest atrocities committed by the Nazi project to exterminate the Jewish people, dying without knowing about the murder of his four sisters in concentration camps. Norbert Elias died on 1 August 1990, a few months after the fall of the Berlin Wall. Despite having lived for more than 90 years, witnessing the transformations of the German State throughout the 20th century, he did not see the outcome of the end of the Cold War or the process of social, political, and economic unification of European nations. Both Freud and Elias, however, were able to foresee, each in their own way, the sufferings that would affect societies and individuals in the coming years.

6.1 A society that demands satisfaction

In 1871, Prussia's victory over the French army led to the formation of the Second Empire of Germany, the *Kaiserreich*, finally allowing Germany to emerge as a great European power. This victory did not only signify a major feat by the military nobility, which led the struggles and further strengthened its position as the representative of the state, but also a defeat for the bourgeoisie that, due to its distancing from military and political issues, had to swap the dream of building a nation unified under liberal, humanist principles for the military values of the aristocracy.

As shown in *The Civilizing Process* (Elias 1939), the distinction between *Kultur* and *Zivilisation* bears an internal contrast of society that ultimately goes back to a national contrast. For the German bourgeoisie, affairs of state were seen as restrictions on any kind of spontaneity of emotions or behaviour. Consequently, the term *Kultur* served to represent the sphere of liberty and equality, situating the bourgeois class in a context outside politics or even as anti-political. For the established nobility, on the other hand, the state was the sphere of coercions and inequalities, as well as the source of their privileges, passed on from generation to generation between aristocratic families. Strictly political behaviour, therefore, was the duty of courtiers who, dominating the forces of the state, promoted nationalist ideas that shaped the true identity of the German people. Furthermore, in Germany, unlike other states, court societies, which held the highest functions of the state, maintained rigid barriers with the bourgeoisie. But, like Freud, Norbert Elias insists on showing us that civilization brings with it its reverse side. Behind the polish, the good manners and the restraint of emotions, what we find is hypocrisy, violence, and the keeping up of appearances.

In his biography of the German State, Elias recalls that between 1871 and 1918 the aristocracy formed what was considered German good society, *die gute Gesellschaft*. One of the criteria for defining what was a good society, he says, was ancestry, family relations between parents and grandparents. The control of the best social positions was therefore passed on via family ties. Old families, normally linked to military tradition, held the monopoly of power and privileges in institutions like the civil service, the army and even universities. Consequently, people who did not have means to access the positions of power and privilege of the high class ended up being stigmatized as outsiders in relation to true society.

In the case of Germany, who unification process came late in comparison with states like France, Spain and Britain, "good societies" were decentralized throughout its extensive geographical territory. No single one predominated over the others. However, as well as family tradition, there was another way of belonging to "good societies". The task of taking on the role of integrating the establishment – composed of Germany's high classes – fell to student groups and their duelling brotherhoods. They instituted, by means of initiation rites, a common code of behaviour marked by the aristocratic custom of the duel and the right to defend one's honour via an armed battle. In this way, individuals could be part of a good society, seeing themselves as superior human beings.

As he did in his research on the civilizing process of the French State, Norbert Elias focused on events and behaviour in the daily life of German individuals. Acceptance into one of the student groups enabled the recognition of the young man as one of "us" in almost all universities in the Reich. His family ties indicated if he was capable of regulating his feelings and behaviour in accordance with the specific codes of the German high class. In this way, it is possible to establish how certain *unsaid* and *unwritten* social rules helped forge the *national habitus* and to mould the personality of the Germans. Elias thus explains this as follows:

> It can be said that these upper classes, different as they were in the many states and cities of Germany, in fact formed a single large society of men who were *satisfaktionsfähig* – able to demand and give satisfaction in a duel. In their social circle, those who enjoyed the privilege of demanding satisfaction with weapon in hand from any other member by whom they felt insulted were obliged in turn to accept the challenge to single combat from fellow members who felt their honour impugned.
>
> (Elias 1989: 51)

With the prospect of a new empire unified under the Kaiser, the German Empire's court society was obliged to open its doors to the bourgeoisie, attracting men from the *intelligentsia*, university professors and civil servants, who ended up adopting this new code of behaviour as a way of including themselves in the aristocratic high class. Among individuals from the bourgeois elite who were rising socially, gradually the balance was swaying towards the codes of behaviour of the higher social class. "The uniform criterion of membership represented by the right to demand or give satisfaction – the recognition of the same code of honour and of single combat", Elias writes, "was certainly not the only sign, but it was the most striking sign, of the formation in German society of a relatively integrated upper class extended by the incorporation of commoners and which was gradually standardised in the wake of the political unification of the *Kaiserreich*" (Elias 1989: 55–56).

For Elias, societies that demanded satisfaction via weapons, whose function was to instil and pass on the codes of norms and emotions of the higher classes, were the touchstone in the construction of a German *national habitus*. The members of the bourgeoisie, who had been raised in a world whose behavioural codes were founded on humanism and equality between people, found themselves living in a world of aristocratic elites whose tradition was rooted in warlike courts and military values. A fusion of standardized sentiments and behaviours with the habits of the most powerful. In this way, in a society where military honour predominated, akin to a *warrior ethos*, establishing a relational logic of the strongest over the weakest, of command and obedience, of domination and subjugation, violence, the symbol of superiority and power, became a fundamental element of the *habitus of the German people*.

Freud's family provides a good example of this situation. A recent publication containing letters exchanged between Sigmund Freud and his children, edited by Michael Schröter, who also edited a number of works by Norbert Elias, like *The Germans*, *Mozart* e *The Society of Individuals*, reveals that Jean-Martin Freud, Freud's eldest son, when he was a child, stood out from the rest of his siblings as the poet of the family. His literary ambitions, however, coexisted with other patterns of behaviour. When he was young, at the time he attended high school and university, he belonged to a Jewish association called Kadimah that practised duels, which allowed him to defend his honour by means of violence. Freud appears to have looked favourably on this, as he himself stated in a letter to his daughter Mathilde: "So far, Oli's Matura and

Martin's Mensur are the biggest sensations" (Freud 2010: 68). Whereas his other son Oliver passed his university entrance exams, Jean-Martin's *Mensur* referred to a kind of initiation duel to join student groups. Jean-Martin became a fencer but, in a contest between Jewish and German students, he ended up being injured.

From 1871 there was an increase of the influence of aristocratic values on the codes of the bourgeoisie, establishing a standardization of rules in a militarized society that demands being honoured. Monarchic codes of behaviour were impacted by the bourgeois makeover of the *warrior ethos*, which imposed itself and rejected the codes that entailed humanist and liberal ideals and aimed to create social equality. As the aristocracy identified itself as the personification of the state, considering itself to be *the* true Germany, this process played an important role in the formation of the German national character. Based on an eminently violent and warlike tradition, rituals and ceremonies ended up serving to establish markers of belonging and of exclusion between the upper and lower classes of society. Elias writes,

> However, the duel also combined the function of differentiating and distancing the higher and lower strata with that of promoting the integration of the higher group itself. Together with their feeling of separation from the lower groups, it reinforced their feeling of belonging to the higher groups and their pride in their membership.
>
> (Elias 1989: 72)

As can be seen, the theory of the configuration between established and outsider groups (Elias 1965) is taken up again in the reading of the German civilizing process. Once again Elias emphasises the interconnectedness between the formation of social structures and the psychic economy of individuals. During the empire of Wilhelm II, and particularly in the two first decades of the 20th century, German court society composed a significant portion of the *satisfaktionsfähige Gesellschaft*. Together with the right to demand satisfaction, the ceremonies, the way of behaving and dressing, the dinners hosted for good society and the physical appearance of residences were symbols of distinction that ultimately served as elements that the high class used to construct an image of themselves as superior human beings, as well as being an attraction for the bourgeois middle class who wishes to climb the social ladder. Elias writes:

> The anchoring of the framework of rules of the *satisfaktionsfdhige Gesellschaft* deep in the individual personality of its members, as a code which has become second nature to them, identifies each individual as belonging to this establishment. His entire habitus – his attitudes, ways of expressing himself, fundamental ideas about human beings, distinguish him as such. That is his reward.
>
> (Elias 1989: 111)

In the case of the student brotherhoods, belonging to a duelling group that had the right to demand satisfaction via use of arms could, above all, be an opportunity to avoid loneliness. Participating in all kinds of social events in university circles, like gatherings, strolls, sporting activities and drunken evenings, created spaces for inclusion for outsider students. Duels and even contests that involved drinking beer in bars served as a means of social distinction that differentiated those who were superior and those who were inferior within this power structure. They gave them courage, honour, discipline, and responsibility, in a process of *romanticization of violence*. Becoming a member of an established group, however, came at a price. It was necessary to adapt yourself psychologically to the demands of the new more traditional, more cohesive and therefore more powerful group. The price of belonging to good society was obeying rules, adapting to etiquette and fulfilling ceremonial traditions, but chiefly being unreservedly subservient to the hierarchy of its most long-standing members.

As Elias always underlines, the individual and society are neither static entities nor separated from each other. Quite the contrary. The drive economy permeates the formation of subjective structures and the formation of social structures, such that we can only think about them as being in a process of differentiated continuity, like two sides of the same coin. The unification of Germany, following victory in the Franco-Prussian war, "there beckoned the hope of escaping from the shadow of a greater past" (Elias 1989: 8), that of the long period of the Holy Roman Empire of the German Nation. With the formation of the Second Empire in 1871 came the possibility of reconstructing a strong, powerful German national identity, also passing on to its citizens the desire to be represented by this same ideal of greatness. In this way, the feelings of weakness and national inferiority were quickly transformed into their opposites, namely feelings of superiority, grandeur and power, sustaining the desire to again become a strong nation and recover supremacy among European states.

The *social myth* of the destiny of a strong, sovereign Germany reappeared with the country's unification in a desire for national hegemony. After many centuries of traumatic experiences, caused by fragmentations and ruptures, by wars and defeats, in turn the Germans could rid themselves of the strong sense of weakness and social inferiority in relation to other European citizens. They could once again fight for a mighty Germany, just as the country had been in its more glorious past. But, as we know, World War I broke out with devastating consequences and with it brought disillusionment, as Freud described in *Thoughts for the Times on War and Death* [*Zeitgemäßes über Krieg und Tod*], of 1915. A text composed of two essays that can be interpreted as the testimonies of a man whose children, family members, colleagues and friends were fighting against foreigners who, despite the ideals of universality and unity among civilized peoples, continued to be assimilated into the concept of enemy. Freud writes:

> Then the war in which we had refused to believe broke out, and it brought – disillusionment. Not only is it more bloody and more destructive than any war of other days, because of the enormously increased perfection of weapons of attack and defence; it is at least as cruel, as embittered, as implacable as any that has preceded it. It disregards all the restrictions known as

> International Law, which in peace-time the states had bound themselves to observe; it ignores the prerogatives of the wounded and the medical service, the distinction between civil and military sections of the population, the claims of private property. It tramples in blind fury on all that comes in its way, as though there were to be no future and no peace among men after it is over. It cuts all the common bonds between the contending peoples, and threatens to leave a legacy of embitterment that will make any renewal of those bonds impossible for a long time to come.
>
> (Freud 1915: 278)

A war was provoked in the name of civilization and a new dimension of psychic trauma was produced along with deaths, waves of mass immigration and the collapse of great empires. The fall of the German Empire and the dissolution of the Austro-Hungarian Empire directly affected both Freud and Elias and the way both of them thought about the world. For Freud, nation-states, sustained by discourses of morality, not only were unable to resolve conflicts but also made their male citizens perpetrators of "deeds of cruelty, fraud, treachery and barbarity so incompatible with their level of civilization that one would have thought them impossible" (1915: 280). A war that broke with any moral or ethical dimension until then upheld as the bulwarks of civilization, making it impossible to renew social ties.

In the same way, Norbert Elias also ponders on this question. The inability to reconcile a highly developed industrial society with mass murder committed by civilized men and women becomes the chief problem to be resolved in *The Germans*. Elias writes,

> Looked at closely, the main problem raised by the mass murder, in the name of a nation, of men, women and children from an alien group, does not lie in the act itself but rather in its incompatibility with the standards which have come to be regarded as distinguishing marks of the most highly developed societies of our time.
>
> (Elias 1989: 302)

It was impossible to believe that such an outbreak of brutality had occurred at the heart of highly civilized modern societies. However, barbarism occurred where civilization existed. The civilizing process is not brought about by "extirpation of evil", but rather by the assimilation of acts of violence that silently remain *unspoken* and suddenly appear as damnable acts. In this same text, Freud positions hypocrisy as the foundation of civilization, a collective fantasy that is produced as an effect of the civilizing process. He thus describes the hypocritical condition as follows:

> Anyone thus compelled to act continually in accordance with precepts which are not the expression of his instinctual inclinations, is living, psychologically speaking, beyond his means, and may objectively be described as a hypocrite, whether he is clearly aware of the incongruity or not. It is

> undeniable that our contemporary civilization favours the production of this form of hypocrisy to an extraordinary extent. One might venture to say that it is built up on such hypocrisy, and that it would have to submit to far-reaching modifications if people were to undertake to live in accordance with psychological truth. Thus there are very many more cultural hypocritesthan truly civilized men – indeed, it is a debatable point whether a certain degree of cultural hypocrisy is not indispensable for the maintenance of civilization, because the susceptibility to culture which has hitherto been organized in the minds of present-day men would perhaps not prove sufficient for the task.
>
> (Freud 1915: 72)

Illusions of grandeur and superiority that are sustained by forgetting one's origins and that are passed on without knowledge of their purpose. But forgetting is not annihilation or extinction. In psychic life, what has been formed does not perish but is preserved and can be brought to light again. If, in 1915, Freud's disillusionment with the uncivilized conduct of citizens and states during the war made him revisit his theory, in 1930, the sense of discontent could no longer refer to disillusionment, nor to unhappiness or discontentment. According the text *Civilization and Its Discontents* [*Das Unbehagen in der Kultur*], civilization does not constantly move towards the future, but shifts between advances and retreats, coming and going, between regressions and evolutions.

In this text of 1930, written in the twilight of dark times, he includes an analysis of the commandment "thou shall love thy neighbour as thyself" as underpinning the ethics of society. Loving one's neighbour as oneself entails impasses and paradoxes of a narcissistic relationship with those like us: if I love a person different to myself, that person must deserve my love, since they are identical to me or to my ideal. But if this is a stranger, why should they receive a portion of my love? A commandment that can only have the function of restricting a natural impulse of human beings. In the formation of alterity, there is always a pull towards its destruction. Thus, Freud echoes the famous utterance of Thomas Hobbes: *homo homini lúpus.* Man is wolf to man. This justifies the existence of commandments that transform aggressive impulses into identifications. The law, however, is not able to promote justice for all, in that it stems from the assimilation of violence.

Under the command of the emperors Wilhelm I and Wilhelm II, grandfather and grandson, the Second Reich did not last for long. World War I occurred and with it another national defeat, another fracturing of the image of superiority that the Germans had constructed of themselves, bringing back the feelings of humiliation, failure and submission. Elias writes:

> For many Germans, the defeat of 1918 was an unexpected, highly traumatic experience. It hit a raw nerve in the national habitus, and was felt to be a return to the time of German weakness, of foreign armies in the country, of a life in the shadow of a greater past.
>
> (Elias 1989: 7)

Good society, which had the right to demand satisfaction, united by a common code of honour and prestige, was once again losing its place in the sun. "A traumatic shock was the consequence" (1989: 183), Elias writes. But not only for the aristocratic class, which had held the power for generations. Equally for the bourgeoisie, which had recently risen socially and had just renounced some of its habits and its values linked to humanism, to freedom of thought and to social equality. The sense of inferiority caused my military defeats in 1918 incited, more than ever, the recovery of the highest values of the German nation.

Consequently, the German civilizing process, according to Elias's thinking, can only be described if the biography of the German State is expanded over the long-term. It is not sufficient to describe internal and external short-term shifts, such as the defeat in the Great War, the economic crisis that devastated the world in the 1920s, the conflicts between the German aristocracy and bourgeoisie caused by power shifts or even a certain penchant for violence allegedly inherent in the behaviour patterns of German citizens. They are in fact fundamental and cannot be excluded from any description of the events that led to the collapse of civilization, as Elias termed the barbarism caused by Hitler.

Alongside these, Elias also references the conflict between older and younger generations, as well as the formation of paramilitary groups, like the *Freikorps*. Made up of soldiers and former officers removed from their posts in the armistice of 1918, these shock troops fought to regain a position of prominence by destroying the parliamentary government that was formed during the Weimar Republic. They were illegal nationalist associations that chiefly used terrorism and acts of violence to re-establish the ideals of aristocratic and military tradition and reconstruct the dream of greatness that underpinned the former German Empire.

Many of the members of the *Freikorps* came to constitute the highest ranks of the National Socialist Party of German Workers [*Nationalsozialistische Deutsche Arbeiterpartei*], such that "The violence of the Nacional Socialist movement", Elias writes, "was, so to speak, the dream of the members of the *Freikorps* and their sympatheizers come true" (Elias 1989: 228). The Nazi officer Reinhard Heydrich, for example, one of the leaders of the SS Central Security Cabinet of the Third Reich, as well as having been one of the chief organizers of the Wannsee Conference, where the final solution to the Jewish question was decided on, at the age of fifteen was part of the first paramilitary organization recognized by the government. It was Heydrich who was responsible for giving Adolf Eichmann, lieutenant-colonel in the SS, the role of planning the logistics of the mass deportation of Jews throughout Europe to the death camps.

Only in this way is it possible to go beyond the conclusions that state that the genocide perpetrated by Hitler was a "cancerous growth on the body of civilized societies", caused by "mentally ill", perverse or immoral people, or even that considered it the consequence of "German traditions and character traits" (Elias 1989: 303). Explanations like these locate barbarism at the opposite pole to civilization, as if it were an exception or an aberration, and reject any possibility of understanding events of this nature as the result of the civilizing process of industrial societies. In opposition to this view, Elias declares: "it might be more fruitful to investigate the conditions in twentieth-century civilizations, the *social* conditions, which have favoured barbarisms of this kind and which might favour them again in the future" (Elias 1989: 303–304).

6.2 The decivilizing spurt

Analysis of the circumstances that led to the decivilizing spurt in Nazi Germany led Norbert Elias to investigate the *social habitus* that shaped a specific personality structure for the German people. His reflections thus began to focus on the social and psychological reasons for the collapse of civilization. In other words, he addressed the following question: what were the circumstances that shaped the German State that over a long period of time weakened the self-control mechanisms of its members, their superegos and their identificatory processes, leading to the genocide of an entire people via the extreme deployment of violence?

Right in the introduction of *The Germans*, Elias underlines some of these circumstances. They are not exclusive to Germany's civilizing process. Other nations-states were also constructed in a similar way. However, according to Elias, "German history over the centuries was, with many ups and downs, a history of decline" (1989: 344). More than the victories and the conquests, what was inscribed in the memory of this people, leaving permanent marks on their *habitus*, in the final analysis, were traumatic events. Difficult to talk about, due to the pain or embarrassment they caused. For a long time people closed their eyes to them, relegating them to silence or oblivion. We must therefore think about the German State as being formed by its catastrophes, its failures, its ruptures and its discontinuities.

Norbert Elias thus highlighted four circumstances that contributed to the construction of a *social habitus* specific to the German people. First, their *geographical location*, within a territory whose borders were constantly changed due to wars with neighbouring countries, as well as causing insecurity for its inhabitants demanded the valorization of military models for conflict resolution. Second, the *elimination struggles*, that took place over centuries between the Germans themselves to attain a higher social position, leaving them weak and powerless to pursue the unification of their state. The victory of the aristocracy, which followed warlike codes, over the *intelligentsia* of the bourgeoisie, underpinned by humanist and egalitarian values, helped create an eminently elitist and military *self-image*. Nationalist values were superimposed on humanist ones. Autocracy won out over democratic policies.

Third, the *breaks* and *discontinuities* affecting the institutions of a state that was unable to coexist without conflicts or wars. The fragility and instability that characterize the German civilizing process created weakened personality structures that were highly dependent on external coercions. Finally, the process by which *militarized aristocratic habitus* were incorporated by wider strata of society gave rise to a nostalgic yearning for a strong leader, a sovereign or a monarch capable of protecting them from themselves and their enemies, in a process that Elias would go on to call *identification with the oppressor*, based on his psychoanalytical studies.

Until 1918, the German social structure was basically organized within an autocratic system, which sanctioned the models of behaviour of the military classes. Within the operational logic of established groups and outsiders, the bourgeoisie sought to merge with the aristocracy, which distinguished itself as a superior group and dominated important functions of the state. It incorporated specific norms and codes specific to the elite class that valorized honour, courage and physical violence. Even the Weimar Republic and the establishment of a more democratic society, with a multi-party parliamentary system, were not enough to disassociate the *social habitus* of the Germans from the *warlike ethos* of the aristocracy nor to change the yearning of the Germans to submit to a sovereign power, a saviour and protector of the nation.

People who were born in societies organized around military codes, like student duelling fraternities and societies that have the right to use armed struggle to get what they want, develop *habitus*, the *second nature* described by Elias, and are more dependent on the commands of leaders. The personality structure of individuals living under an authoritarian state thus becomes relatively simple. They do not have to deal with conflicts, divergences, differences, or contradictions, as is the case in democratic, multi-party states. They merely have to obey the orders from above. Elias writes,

> A personality structure attuned to an absolutist-monarchic or dictatorial regime allows great scope for a readiness in the individual person to accept orders, to allow him- or herself to be guided by external constraints. The individual citizen is then spared the heavy burden of having to participate in debates with people of different opinions. The ruled do not need to decide in favour of one side or the other. The order comes from above; the decision has been made.
>
> (1989: 291)

The personality structure of the Germans was therefore being slowly constructed from an eminently authoritarian tradition, underpinned by an operational logic of obedience to orders. Consequently, affective relationships ended up reproducing the positions of *those who give orders* and *those who obey*, supporting the desire of individuals to be controlled by a strong leader and to live under rigid social norms. Elias thus continues,

> Under a regime of this type, the individual person still remains in a child-like status in relation to the state. Parental orders are certainly not always comfortable, and the same is also true of the orders of aristocratic princes and dictators. But in the end one trusts them. And if one does not obey, the military or the police, which are among the main pillars of the organization of a monolithic autocratic state, will quickly step into action.
>
> (Elias 1989: 261)

For Germans, the imperative was categorical. The close dependency on an autocratic form of government passed on unstable standards of self-control linked to a sovereign power that externally exercises control over his impulses, desires, behaviour and own autonomy of thought. Thus, Elias writes, there is an adjustment between the personality structures and the political structures. The Germans refused to reflect in the image that they constructed of themselves the histories of their own country's failures and defeats, exaggerating their greatness and superiority. A selective memory that emphasized the great feats of the nation's history and repressed in the depths of psychic life feelings of inferiority, weakness and shame.

According to Elias, "The image of a nation experienced by an individual who forms part of that nation, therefore, is also a constituent of that person's self-image. The virtue, the value, the meaningfulness of the nation are also his or her own" (Elias 1989: 151–152). A process of identification that does not separate or distinguish between the terms individual and state but considers them as intrinsically connected entities. Pride and valorization of the German nation, expressed in nationalism and patriotism, were hyperbolic feelings based on collective fantasies that sought, in a national ideal, what was lacking in reality. For Norbert Elias, *nationalism* is "a social belief system which, latently or acutely, raises the state-society, the sovereign collectivity to which its members belong, to the position of a supreme value to which all other values can and sometimes must be subordinated" (Elias 1989: 153–154). The manipulation of emotions by states and societies, governments and political regimes, is a recurrent technique used to shape a particular personality structure. A school's educational process or the way social memories are preserved and passed on, for example, are profoundly affected by political ideologies and beliefs focused on the interests of the most powerful groups.

German vainglory, in this sense, also projected its shadows. The Germans rarely felt they matched up to the ideals they constructed of themselves: "The German national ideal was like a brilliant star high up in the sky" (Elias 1989: 326), as Elias writes. In fact, an idealism that took the lead, and attributed value and meaning also demanded loyalty, sacrifice and submission from individuals. Expressed via patriotism or nationalism, it presented itself as a form of *collective egoism* that, as Freud described in relation to how the masses function, served to affirm the narcissisms of identities and antagonize the differences of outsider groups. In the text *Group Psychology and the Analysis of the Ego* (Freud 1921), Freud showed that the love that the individual displaces onto a collective entity is nothing more than self-love displaced onto another object. In Elias's words we find a formulation that is very close to Freud's idea:

> The love for one's nation is never only a love for persons or groups of whom one says "you"; it is always also the love of a collectivity to which one can refer as "we". Whatever else it may be, it is also a form of self-love.
>
> (Elias 1989: 151)

The identity of every individual is intimately linked to the identity of the groups he belongs to and the reinforcement of the "we" identity is therefore remains a way of distinguishing and excluding other identities.

Emotions that shape representations of oneself, *self-images*, also permeate collective representations, *we-images*, such that the love individuals have for their nation is also the expression of the love they have for themselves. A form of self-love that fixes the *self-image* and the *self-ideal* to the *we-image* and *we-ideal*. The *self-ideal* tells each individual what he is, what he should do and how he should be and behave, always in accordance with the *we-ideal* that he belongs to. Aggression and destructiveness, that many deemed to be characteristics of the nature of the German people, Elias writes, were above all the expression of a *social habitus* that required that individuals used physical force, violence, and virility whenever their *we-ideals* demanded for the sake of Germany. A national ideal transmitted, taught and learned, that expected the destruction of anyone considered a threat to national sovereignty.

In the view of Norbert Elias, therefore, we cannot understand the National Socialism, which led Hitler's Germany to try to decimate an entire people, without taking into consideration the long-term social process that led to the rigid, inflexible and absolute idealism of national beliefs. The collapse of civilization can thus only be understood in terms of the total dedication of the Germans to their *we-ideal*. Collective values unconditionally prevail over individual ones, even if they contradict the ethical and moral principles that regulate civilized relations.

As previously stated, the theory about the configurations between established groups and outsider ones was essential for Elias's development of his analyses of the German decivilizing process. The pride and honour in being part of an aristocratic group that considered itself superior because it followed patterns of control imposed by the state, like external coercions [*Fremdzwang*], produced within individuals' patterns of control, internal coercions [*Selbstzwang*], more attuned to and dependent on the idea of being governed from above. Belonging to the organisation of the state, being part of the privileged class of the German aristocracy, was a way of sharing the sense of "us" as opposed to the "them" of the bourgeois classes and the masses, but also of finding value and meaning for one's own life. Consequently, the German "us" was much more focused on the idea of an autocratic system, whose central power was concentrated in a strong leader, one man capable of maintaining order and discipline. The oppressive nature of the authority of the state thus matched the interior voices of the Germans via the formation of *we-ideals*.

More individualistic societies usually find a meaning to life in the relationship between individuals. Without other people, without the role they have on us, it is not possible to create a life with purpose. This occurs in various ways. A profession, wealth inherited from a birth family, belonging to the military, a religion, even owning a stamp collection or the unconditional love for a child, Elias states, enable people's lives to have meaning, constructing their own identity linked to the group they belong to. In the case of the Germans, this *invisible link*, that creates a collective identity and joins individuals to each other, was intrinsically part of their relationship with Germany. Each individual's *self-image* silently contains the image of his nation. A national consciousness that reflects national ideals, interweaving national, intra- and inter-state levels.

As was the case in Norbert Elias's analyses of court societies, where the social dynamic of the French court was connected to the dynamic of psychic structures, in German society the threats the state faced from internal or external enemies are considered a threat to the very identity of individuals. But not just that. The loss of a social position of superiority and sovereignty for those who are seen as foreigners, marginals, or outsiders, could affect one's self-love and pride and even put one's life in danger. The traumatic process of the formation of the German State, which took place during a slow decline over centuries and centuries, gradually shaped a specific personality for the German people that generated specific *social habitus* for its members and a weakened, diminished, and insecure personality of itself.

> If a process of decline takes place slowly, if the struggle to bring it to a halt stretches over the generations and remains undecided for a long time, if occasional upturns and recoveries from time to time rekindle hopes for the restoration of the old glory, if, in short, the decline never goes so far that people *have* to face up to it, then the ambiguities of a nation's status and the symptoms of a massive status-insecurity can sink deep into the make-up of its members and permeate their entire tradition of beliefs and conduct. This is precisely what happened in the case of the development of Germany.
>
> (Elias 1989: 359)

In the case of the Germans, whose history is marked by traumatic experiences, this shock causes fragmentations in their personalities. The feelings of disillusionment, discouragement, lack of self-worth, self-depreciation, inadequacy, and lack of purpose in life were then transformed into their superlative opposites. Courage, fearlessness and bravura, self-confidence, autonomy and determination, virtue, and honour finally became defining character traits of the Germans. This was combined with the formation of rigid, inflexible national beliefs, national ideals that sought in the stories of the past a glory that was not materializing in the present and the desire to transform Germany into an entity that ruled over Europe and the rest of the world. A national belief that aimed to make them feel that they belonged to humanity's elite. The atrocities and barbaric acts committed against the Jews, supported by the ideology of the purity of the German race, thus became a further attempt to restore the greatness and superiority of that nation. Even those people who felt inferior were able to think and behave in a barbaric, cruel way, far removed from the civilizing principles they had been brought up with.

The German decivilizing process led by the Nazis was in part the result of the threats they felt as they tried to realize their ambition to make Germany a great world power again, something their national ideals had dreamed of. However, the predominance of the *we-ideal* over the *self-ideal* does not adequately explain the decivilizing impetus and the eruption of barbarism during the Third Reich. Many groups and nations also hold, as expressed in patriotism and nationalism, feelings of loyalty, and duty embedded within all individuals in the form of the *we-ideal*. Norbert Elias therefore gives a more in-depth meta-psychological reading of the formation of the German *social habitus* recognizing in the *identification with the oppressor* [*Identifizierung mit dem Unterdrücker*] a psychological process characteristic of the German people, essential for understanding the decivilizing impetus that led regression of civilization under the Third Reich.

6.3 The metapsychology of the decivilizing process

Norbert Elias was initially influenced by psychoanalysis in the early 1930s, when he was still Karl Mannheim's assistant, in the Sociology Department at the University of Frankfurt, where he had close contact with the researchers of the well-known *Frankfurt School*. During the time he lived in England, Anna Freud's psychoanalytical current, also known as *Ego Psychology*, was one of the main theoretical references for those close to him, which included his own analyst, Kate Friedlander, and his colleague and friend Siegmund Foulkes, one of the co-founders, with Elias, of the Group Analytic Society.

Although recognizing something traumatic in the constitution of the psyche, the *identification with the aggressor* described by Anna Freud is considered one of the normal defence mechanisms for the constitution of morality. In her book *The Ego and the Mechanisms of Defence*, Anna Freud presents *identification with the aggressor* as a normal development process of the superego. According to her, via the shift from a position of passivity to one of activity, the child identifies with characteristics of an adult who caused them anxiety as a way of assimilating the unpleasant experience they have just gone through. A process that had already been described by her father in the text *Beyond the Pleasure Principle* (Freud 1920). Observing his grandson playing, Sigmund Freud noticed that the child elaborated the anxiety caused by separation from his mother by reproducing the movement of making a cotton reel appear and disappear underneath the sofa. Behaviour that was accompanied by the exclamation *o-o-o-o*, when the object went away from him, a way of trying to say the word *Fort!* ("far", "absent"), and, joyfully, by the utterance *Da!* ("here", "over there"), when he could see the object again.

For Anna Freud (1936), *identification with the aggressor* personifies an aggressor as a way of lessening the anxiety caused by a violent situation. Via this defence mechanism, the child ceases to be threatened and becomes the one who is threatening. They internalize the aggression coming from the outside world and, before transferring it to themselves, in the form of a feeling of guilt, they project outwardly the same aggressivity that they were on the receiving end of. Anna Freud writes,

> An ego which with the aid of the defense mechanism of projection develops along this particular line introjects the authorities to whose criticism it is exposed and incorporates them in the superego. It is then able to project the prohibited impulses outward. Its intolerance of other people precedes its severity toward itself. It learns what is regarded as blameworthy but protects itself by means of this defense mechanism from unpleasant self-criticism.
>
> (Freud 1936: 119)

Anna Freud situates *identification with the aggressor* as a preliminary phase in the establishment of the superego and morality, part of a normal process in the constitution of the psyche. Via this defence mechanism, therefore, we cannot distinguish any specific formation of personality that would help us answer the question "what is it to be German?" and thus obtain a different answer to the questions "what is it to be French?" or "what is it to be English?". Furthermore, Anna Freud appears not to consider socio-historical contexts that permeate the formation of psychic structures, reducing *identification with the aggressor*, ultimately, to an intrapsychic operation that extends, at most, to the most familiar relationships. For Norbert Elias, and he underlines this point, the formation of the German *social habitus* should be described as a response to the succession of traumatic experiences that permeated the civilizing process of Germany over the centuries.

As we know, since its beginnings, Freudian theory attributed importance to traumatic causality. First, in the overall theory of seduction, abandoned almost immediately to make way for oedipal sexual fantasies. Then, traumatic neuroses produced in the context of the Great War returned to the importance of society in the development of psychic illness. Finally, from 1920, the discovery of the death drive and repetition compulsion revealed themselves as human beings' silent, natural tendency towards destruction. Via the death drive, Freud (1933) tried to explain war as a destiny, even an inevitable one, of the civilizing process. His drive theory, however, also does not seem to adequately help us understand the socio-historical context that led Hitler's Germany to reverse civilization in the direction of barbarism. It is necessary to go beyond Sigmund Freud, and also his daughter, and examine another psychoanalytical theory to find some openings for dialoguing with the meta-psychological hypotheses of Norbert Elias in relation to the formation of the German people's personality.

The dialogue between the concept of *identification with the oppressor*, as it was presented by Elias, and the concept of *identification with the aggressor*, developed by the Hungarian psychoanalyst Sándor Ferenczi, helps us to understand the metapsychology of the German decivilizing process. Bringing these two concepts together may seem odd and even unsettling to some, especially those who restrict themselves to theoretical purisms. As far as I am aware, Elias never made any kind of reference to Sándor Ferenczi in his texts or interviews and, as far as I have been able to discover in my research, there is no publication that relates the two authors to each other. Nevertheless, I take on board Juan Tuber-Oklander's (2019) suggestion that Ferenczi silently influenced the origin and the development of group psychoanalysis. In his view there is exchange and a mutual influence between individual processes and collective ones, narrowing the relationship between psychic structures and social ones and seeking to go beyond the antithesis between "individual *versus* society". Furthermore, the psychoanalyst S. H. Foulkes (1937), one of the founders of the *Group Analytic Society* together with Norbert Elias, focused on the differences between the concepts of introjection, identification, and projection in Ferenczi's work.

Like Norbert Elias, Sándor Ferenczi was and still is an author whose importance has been devalued and, it is fair to say, even dismissed by the psychoanalytic community. Born in Hungary and a graduate in medicine from the University of Vienna, Ferenczi was one of the first and closest disciples of Sigmund Freud. He served on the front as a doctor in the Hungarian army during World War I and for years studied the psychic suffering of former combatants. He died in 1933 and did not live to witness the barbaric acts committed by the Nazis. But it was, in fact, from treating patients with issues relating to their identificatory processes that he was able to pass on to the field of psychoanalysis the importance of social and political relations in the production of traumatic experiences. From Ferenczi's work, therefore, psychoanalysis began to make significant contributions to the field of social trauma. Maria Torok writes about Ferenczi's oeuvre in its entirety as follows:

> If someone asked me to summarize in a word the entire subject matter of Ferenczi's work, it would be this one [catastrophe] and its synonyms: traumas, accidents, diseases, pathos. In the same way, if I had to name the keystone around which psychoanalytic quarrels revolve it would still be the word catastrophe.
>
> (Torok 2001: 81)

Following the similarities between his ideas and Freud's, in 1908, there were many texts in which Ferenczi highlighted the importance of the social and family context in the formation of mental illness. From the late 1920s, however, the *enfant terrible* of psychoanalysis, with his restless, questioning mind, began specializing in the treatment of patients considered difficult, dealing increasingly often with the question of pathogenic trauma. At that time, Ferenczi wrote books like *The Adaptation of the Family to the Child* [*Die Anpassung der Familie na das Kind*], of 1928, and *The Unwelcome Child and his Death Instinct* [*Das unwillkommene Kind und sein Todestrieb*], of 1929, where he considered trauma as experiences that require a child to adapt their behaviour to be part of society. He lists the following events: "the traumata of weaning, training to cleanliness, the breaking of 'bad habits', and, last and most important of all, the breaking off from childhood itself into the adult way of life" (Ferenczi 1928: 59).

Nevertheless, from the 1930s, texts appeared like *The Principle of Relaxion and Neocatharsis* [*Relaxationprinzip und Neokatharsis*], of 1930, and *Child Analysis in the Analysis of Adults* [*Kinderanalysen mit Erwachsenen*], of 1931, where Ferenczi began to describe trauma as an effect of a violent shock on a totally vulnerable and unprepared individual. He went into more detail about his trauma theory in at least three other texts, as follows: *Confusion on Tongues between the Adults and the Children* [*Sprachverwirrung zwischen den Erwachsenen und dem Kind. Die Sprache der Zärtllichkeit umd der Leidenschaft*], of 1932, *Some Thoughts on Trauma* [*Gedanken über das Trauma*], published posthumously in 1934, and his *The Clinical Diary of Sándor Ferenczi*, written in 1932 and published in 1969, over three decades after his death.

What leads us to return to the ideas of Sándor Ferenczi, at this point, is his definition of the concept of *identification with the aggressor*, constructed from a new theory on trauma. Instead of referring to a normal process of the constitution of the superego, like Anna Freud, Ferenczi argues that *identification with the aggressor* is directly bound up with the experiences of violence that occur within social relationships. It is necessary, therefore, to start with the way he thinks about the social condition of psychic trauma, especially in his texts from the 1930s. To summarize, we can say that for Ferenczi, if the experience of violence has no possibility of being enunciated, it inscribes itself in individuals as social trauma. In other words, the lack of social recognition about the testimony of a traumatic experience is capable of causing a kind of rupture, or even annihilation, of psychic life.

Trauma thus ceases to be constitutive for individuals and is now considered in terms of its pathogenic value, occurring necessarily at two separate moments. In the first, which we can call the *shock*, a real event has an overwhelming impact on the individual. The shock occurs suddenly, unexpectedly, out of nowhere, and unpredictably. Normally the individual is caught unawares. Ferenczi describes the precondition for a traumatic experience:

> Shock always comes upon one *unprepared*. It must needs be preceded by a feeling of *security*, in which, because of the subsequent events, one feels *deceived*; one trusted in the *external world too much* before; after, too little or not at all. One had to have overestimated one's own powers and to have lived under the delusion that *such things* could not happen, not *to me*.
>
> (Ferenczi 1932a: 230 – emphasis in original)

The individual's trust in the context and in their surroundings gives rise to the belief that nothing bad could happen to them, leaving them unprepared for the most excessive situations. Consequently, when the worst happens, they are always caught off-guard. A situation that could easily be avoided. As Ferenczi writes in his *Clinical Diary*: "Immediately after the events (generally in childhood) the victim of the shock could still have been helped" (Ferenczi 1932b: 25). The individual who has suffered the first shock could still be saved, since the encounter with the other, he argues, facilitates the elaboration of this violence: "One gets the impression that children get over even severe shocks without amnesia or neurotic consequences, if the mother is at hand with understanding and tenderness and (what is most rare) with complete sincerity" (Ferenczi 1931: 125). Ferenczi contends that it is enough for the other to be present, recognizing that the violent experience actually occurred, acknowledging the suffering and the individual's truth.

The individual who suffered a shock is reduced to a complete state of passivity, accepting everything without resistance. "An unexpected, unprepared for, overwhelming shock acts like, as if it were, an anaesthetic" (Ferenczi 1932a: 218), Ferenczi writes. They suspend any kind of psychic activity, in a paralysis that includes the suspension of motility, perception and thought. The shock thus amounts, according to Ferenczi, to the "annihilation of self-regard, of the ability to put up a resistance, and to act and think in defence of one's own self" (1932a: 230). In other words, after the shock, the individual becomes incapable of producing any reaction. They cannot even perceive sensible reality, what is right before their eyes. They do not even recognize evil, especially that caused by moral suffering.

An external threat, the meaning of which cannot be grasped, Ferenczi writes, is unbearable. In his *Clinical Diary*, he states,

> If a trauma strikes the soul, or the body, unprepared, that is, with- out countercathexis, then its effect is destructive for body and mind, that is, it disrupts through fragmentation. The power that would hold the individual fragments and elements together is absent.
>
> (Ferenczi 1932b: 69)

The only possibility of escaping from this situation is self-destruction, the annihilation of what maintains the cohesion of the psychic formations in entity. As a result, what we find following the shock is a psychic disorientation, a destroyed, decomposed personality, made up of ruins and fragments.

Furthermore, as a consequence of the shock, "no memory traces of such impressions remain, even in the unconscious, and thus the causes of the trauma cannot be recalled from memory traces" (Ferenczi 1932a: 218). Everything occurs as if the trauma was surrounded by a retroactive amnesia. In a traumatic experience,

> a part of our personality can "die", and if the remaining part does survive the trauma, it wakes up with a gap in its memory, actually with a gap in the personality, since it is not just the memory of the death struggle that has selectively disappeared or perhaps has been destroyed, but all the associations connected with it as well.
>
> (Ferenczi 1932b: 179)

The first moment of the trauma, however, is not sufficient to render the experience pathogenic. At that point, Ferenczi introduces a fundamental point from which he moves away from Freudian theory. The trauma is not a factor *sine qua non* of the psychic constitution of individuals, as Freud (1926) posited, even making reference to the trauma of birth as paradigmatic of this experience. In Ferenczi's view, trauma is the result of a relational context. In this sense, Ferenczi is considered a precursor of object relations theory.

The second moment of the trauma is that of *the denial*. At this point the truth of a violence suffered by someone is denied by other individuals. The child that experienced a shock is unable to immediately recount, easily and precisely, what has happened to them. Still confused, they seek out an adult to be able to pass the experience on and confirm that the suffering that they have gone through actually happened. This other individual must be someone they can trust, a person able to believe what they are being told. However, if the account of the violent experience is not acknowledged by the other person as true, the child ends up being silenced in a traumatic way. The trauma does not therefore lie in the intensity of the shock itself, nor in its resignification *a priori*, as Freud had proposed, but in the social interdiction of the individual's possibilities to express their own experience.

In his theory about trauma, Ferenczi stresses the social nature of its formation. In his opinion, there are several ways that individuals can react when presented with a narrative of violence. With incomprehension, with punishment or a deathly silence. Normally the episode is received as if nothing has happened. But Ferenczi underlines that the denial that becomes the pathogenic trauma can also demand of the individual *heroism* towards a situation that they cannot deal with alone. The Hungarian expression *katonadolog* demands from the child a degree of heroism that he is not yet capable of. This is equivalent to the expression "soldiers can take it", that ignores the vulnerability of the child, isolating them from relationships with others and forcing them to cope alone in the face of a greater force.

> In most cases of infantile trauma, the parents have no interest in impressing the events on the mind of the child, on the contrary, the usual cure is repression: "it's nothing at all"; "nothing has happened"; "don't think about it"; "katonadolog"; but nothing is ever said about these ugly matters (for instance of a sexual nature). Such things are simply hidden in a deadly silence; the child's faint references are ignored or even rejected as incongruous, with the unanimous concurrence of those around him, and with such consistency that the child has to give up and cannot maintain its own judgment.
>
> (Ferenczi 1932b: 25)

In the constitution of a trauma, the lack of acknowledgement rebounds not only on the truth of the testimony of the violent event, but above all on the very individual who has related it. Thus, in the text *The Child Analysis in the Analysis of Adult*, Ferenczi describes the way that the second moment of the trauma begins:

> Probably the worst way of dealing with such situations is to deny their existence, to assert that nothing has happened and that nothing is hurting the child. Sometimes he is actually beaten or scolded when he manifests traumatic paralysis of thought and movement. These are the kinds of treatment which make the trauma pathogenic.
>
> (Ferenczi 1931: 125)

In German, the term used by Ferenczi is *Verleugnung*, commonly translated in Freud's work as denial, disavowal or abnegation. This concept was coined by Freud and has been given different meanings in his theorization. But it was above all as a description of the defence mechanism of perversions that it came to prominence, even leading him to have to revise his theory of civilization. In his text about fetishism (Freud 1927), where he states that a fetish is constructed via the *abnegation of reality* (the reality of castration), denial is differentiated from the repression [*Verdrängung*] of neurosis and from the rejection [*Verwerfung*] of psychosis.

Denial does not mean ignoring or repressing castration but being able to simultaneously have two contradictory thoughts. Within denial *knowing* and *not knowing* a reality coexist. Eleven years later, Freud (1940) wrote the text *Splitting of the Ego in the Process of Defence* [*Die Ichspaltung im Abwehrvorgang*]. Unfinished, due to his death, the concept of denial is returned to in order to explain the particular process of withdrawal of the individual from reality, without them falling into psychosis. What happens, according to Freud, is a *cleavage of the ego* in which one part, faced with the possibility of suffering a psychic trauma, does not recognize reality, whereas the other affirms its existence.

What we see in Freud's work is the description of an intrapsychic process in which the ego is fractured when faced with the possibility of an unbearable traumatic experience. The ego's function of synthetic unity thus ceases to be a regulating principle. In *Moses and the Monotheism* (Freud 1939), denial serves to explain the way that the civilizing process deals with examples of violence and experiences of catastrophes. In this way societies seek to eliminate the signs of a truth just like, at a crime scene, the criminal tries to make all traces of himself disappear. Denial and psychic cleavage thus take on a social dimension.

There are few similarities between Ferenczi's and Freud's descriptions of denial. For the Hungarian psychoanalyst, this mechanism is a response caused by a third-party who silences language in their representative attributions, treating the traumatic experience as if it had not happened. More than the shock, it is the denial that causes the trauma. In his *Clinical Diary*, to the question, "What is traumatic: an attack or its consequence?", Ferenczi answers: "Traumatic confusion arises mainly because the attack and the response to it are denied by the guilt-ridden adults, indeed, are treated as deserving punishment" (1932b: 178). When met with denial, the individual's perceptions are invalidated, their truth is relegated to the level of lie and their words are completely stripped of authority. Denial strips the individual of their spaces of enunciation, paralyses the spontaneity of their thoughts, removes their will to live and abandons them in a state of vulnerability.

"Oh, it is only a child, he does not know anything, he will forget it all" (Ferenczi 1933: 147). These could be the words of an adult seducer who does not believe that their violence can cause any kind of harm to an abused child. But this same logic of reasoning can also be repeated by a society, when it does not recognize violence that affects its population. Denial does in fact lead to forgetting. But forgetting does not mean eliminating, nor making something disappear. Denial causes a hole in one's memory, which also impacts on all associated memories, preventing the formation of links between one event and another. It inscribes gaps in the chain of recollections, it jumbles references and interrupts narrative sequences from which the individual constructs their identity. For Ferenczi, the contestation of the reality of an experience by someone who should be and should give support, obliges the individual to deny not just what they felt, perceived and understood, but also their very existence.

The way Sándor Ferenczi describes the moments of trauma seems very similar to Norbert Elias's understanding of the specificity of the development of the German civilizing process and the particular way the personality of the German people was constructed. For Elias, there was, and in some sense there still is in Germany, a policy of banning public discussions about painful social events. A stance of disregard for the past that believes that "it would be possible to continue to pursue the business of Germany as though nothing had happened, and that the best thing for the German people would be to forget the National Socialist interlude", says Elias, which led the Germans to believe that "they believed they could draw a line under the past" (Elias 1989: 431).

The German State was thus shaped by a succession of denials [*Verleugnung*] about collective traumatic experiences that, relegated to oblivion, penetrated deep into the psychic economy of its members, causing serious damage to their personalities. The catastrophes, fragmentations and discontinuities suffered by the Germans, repressed and denied over century after century, gradually created fractured personalities, rupturing the identity of the German people, and causing cracks in their *self-image.*

As a consequence of denial, there is a process that Ferenczi terms *narcissistic cleavage.* Ferenczi uses some images to explain this process. In one of them, he says that the traumatised individual reacts like a worm-eaten fruit: "It is natural to compare this with the precocious maturity of the fruit that was injured by a bird or insect" (Ferenczi 1933: 149). A part of the fruit is ripe on the outside and another part is destroyed in the middle. A ripeness or maturity that is hastily acquired in an attempt to overcome the suffering caused by violence.

Another image that Ferenczi uses to describe the effects of psychic cleavage is taken from one of his dreams. Ferenczi writes: "I wish to remind you of the typical 'dream of the wise baby' described by me several years ago in which a newly-born child or an infant begins to talk, in fact teaches wisdom to the entire family" (Ferenczi 1933: 149). The ego thus divides into a sensitive part, brutally destroyed, whereas the other part, in a way, knows everything but feels nothing. One part carries with it a twin that was inhibited, whereas the other part, which was spared, is responsible for adapting to reality. The child matures more quickly than its years. It is as if the individual's personality had been "kidnapped from itself".

A state of self-alienation, in which the individual, on forgetting themselves, manages to maintain the illusion of protection when faced with the external world. In psychic cleavage, therefore, there is a dual movement of progression and regression. This is the mechanism that Ferenczi goes on to call "traumatic progression". While one part of the individual's personality regresses to a pre-traumatic time, seeking to annul the event that caused the shock, at the same time the other part progresses towards a state of maturity, civility and edification. In his *Clinical Diary*, Ferenczi writes,

> What is new in this whole process is that in addition to the flight from reality in the regressive sense there is also. a flight in a progressive sense, a sudden development of intelligence, even clairvoyance – that is, a progressive flight, a sudden flowering of developmental possibilities virtually present in outline but hitherto functionally not utilized.
>
> (Ferenczi 1932b: 203)

This explains, one can argue, Norbert Elias's description of the ambivalences of the civilizing process of the German people and how societies that have attained high levels of civilisation are able to intentionally commit barbaric acts that go against the fundamental principles on which they are built. Precocious maturity, the sudden acquisition of an adult knowledge, or even the progress of civilization can actually mask a reaction to a traumatic denial at the heart of social relations.

The ego divides into a superstructure that maintains the highest moral values and corresponds to the highest standards of civilization, super-intellectualized and with high levels of self-control of drives, and an infrastructure that is primitive and intensely emotional, extremely dependent on external controls. Consequently, Ferenczi writes, object relations, that have become impossible, are transformed into narcissistic relations in an attempt to cancel out the abandonment of the trauma, as occurs with "the man abandoned by all gods":

> The man abandoned by all gods escapes completely from reality and creates for himself another world in which he, unimpeded by earthly gravity, can achieve everything that he wants. Has he been unloved, even tormented, he now splits off from himself a part which in the form of a helpful, loving, often motherly, minder commiserates with the tormented remainder of the self, nurses him and decides for him; and all this is done with deepest wisdom and most penetrating intelligence. He is intelligence and kindness itself, so to speak a guardian angel. This angel sees the suffering or murdered child from the outside (consequently he must have, as it were, escaped out of the person in the process of 'bursting'), he wanders through the whole Universe seeking help, invents fantasies for the child that cannot be saved in any other way, etc.
>
> (Ferenczi 1932a: 216)

Ferenczi's description refers to a weakened personality exclusively made up of the id and superego. The processes of identification between the *ego ideal* and the *we-ideal* cease to take place via the mediation of the ego and cease to be products of the repression of drives and emotions, as described by the civilizing process. Via a kind of mimesis, individuals' identifications with collective ideals now represent narcissistic interests of the part of the personality that was traumatized. Ferenczi writes, in his *Clinical Diary*: "a part of her person gets 'beside itself'; the area thus vacated is filled by the will of what has terrified her" (Ferenczi 1932b: 48) and further on he states: "the evil in people lives on, as it were, in the minds of those who have been ill treated" (Ferenczi 1932a: 59). This internalized aggressor, that has invaded and taken possession of the personality of traumatized individuals, is no longer the representative of paternal authority, but a sadistic and tyrannical superego that usurps the singular conditions of representation, invalidates the pluralities of significations and silences the spaces of enunciation. This ideal submits the traumatized individual to the authority of its unequivocal, unquestionable and absolute truth.

Ferenczi then describes another consequence of this psychic schism. It is the process of *identification with the aggressor*, a concept that Norbert Elias takes from psychoanalysis to think about the imbrication between the autocracy of the German State – based on a central power concentrated in a strong man, who passed on models of behaviour specific to the military classes and installed unstable standards of self-control, more dependent on external coercions – and the metapsychology of the personality structure of the German people.

The child, in its vulnerability, feeling physically and morally defenceless, with a personality that is still too fragile to defend itself against the force of an authority, submits to the will of the aggressor, forgets themselves, and identifies totally with that aggressor. Ferenczi writes:

> The same anxiety, however, if it reaches a certain maximum, compels them to subordinate themselves like automata to the will of the aggressor, to divine each one of his desires and to gratify these; completely oblivious of themselves they identify themselves with the aggressor.
>
> (1933: 146)

For the child who has been violated, it is safer to identify with the person who attacked them than to lose their love and protection. Ferenczi continues: "Through the identification, or let us say, introjection of the aggressor, he disappears as part of the external reality, and becomes intra- instead of extra-psyche" (1933: 146). The aggressor invades the childlike a squatter, taking control of their ego, or part of it.

In this way, individuals end up taking up more submissive and obedient positions, are inclined to identify with other people, forgetting about their own wills, feelings and desires. "The misused child changes into a mechanical, obedient automaton or becomes defiant, but is unable to account for the reasons of his defiance" (1933: 147), Ferenczi writes. A masochism that leaves them paralyzed, incapable of reacting to displeasure or even of constructing more creative responses to break with rigidly established social relations. The states of passivity, obedience, submission and silencing are reinforced by the introjection of a feeling of guilt caused by the aggressor.

According to Ferenczi, acts of violence are normally accompanied by a certain morality, coldness and shame on the part of their perpetrator. "Not infrequently after such events, the seducer becomes over-moralistic or religious and endeavours to save the soul of the child by severity" (Ferenczi 1933: 147). The introjected feeling of guilt leads the individual to repeat the traumatic scene in their most varied relationships, reproducing emotional ties organized in accordance with an identificatory model that establishes asymmetrical positions between, on the one hand, the supreme power, the aggressor, the dominator, and on the other the victim, the tyrannized, the submissive and the dominated.

Up to now we have been exploring the concept of *identification with the aggressor*, in the form that Ferenczi presented it, in order to understand how Norbert Elias returned to the metapsychology of *identification with the oppressor* in the formation of the personality structures of Germans. According to Elias, the history of Germany was marked by a series of catastrophes and tragedies that penetrated deeply the psychic economy of members of that nation. An autocratic state ruled by a supreme power that controlled individuals from top to bottom and demanded of them submission to rigorous rules and regulations, an absolute obedience to any national duty whatsoever. Gradually the value of the *self-image* of Germans was directly linked to the value of the image that they built of their nation. The *ego ideal* of Germans was being surrendered to the *we-ideal* of Germany. In addition, the level of external control exerted by the state created *social habitus* integrated into national codes.

The German State, as Elias describes, was becoming an oppressor to its members. Its values, ideals, codes and rules were internalized, but in such a way that individuals had no autonomy to manage their emotions, their behaviour and their thoughts. "It was this dependency which gave the German identification with nation and state – and if the state was oppressive, with the oppressor – its specific stamp" (1989: 386), Elias writes. The autocratic, absolutist German State had a control over individuals that caused a conflict between the desire for personal survival and the desire for survival of the nation. However, there was not really a choice. Individuals were coerced into submitting to the nation. A "desire for submission" thus established itself as a tendency among Germans, who subordinated themselves, often willingly and enthusiastically, to authority, to a strong leader or ruler who represented the ideals of the nation.

Norbert Elias explains as follows:

> When rule is autocratic and when, as was normally the case in the past and still is in many societies today, it is merely exercised primarily for the benefit of the rulers and more or less oppressively, the adherence in thinking, feeling and acting to the common national creed does, in fact, have the character of an identification with the oppressors.
>
> (Elias 1989: 377–378)

Norbert Elias recognizes a satisfaction in the Germans' obedience to the demands of the state. In fact, obedience and submission are reinforced by internalized voices, as Elias states:

> Above all in times of crisis, people are driven through reciprocal reinforcements more and more to exaggerate the demands of their "inner voices", their beliefs and convictions, their moral principles, ideals or whatever, and to obey them more and more uncompromisingly.
>
> (Elias 1989: 343).

The ego, as Freud describe, feels satisfied when it manages to fulfil the orders and obligations imposed by the superego. It feels that it has attained the level of the *ego ideal* and that it is deserving of the love of this protective entity. However, in the case of the Germans, we must remember that this superego represents an oppressor, in the face of which the ego assumes its *desire for submission*. The satisfaction of submitting thus merely represents a traumatized personality, that only manages to keep itself alive if it assumes unquestioning obedience.

There is nothing more traumatic for an individual than the destruction of the values and meanings of their life. When people's lives seem to depend, ultimately, on the preservation of their nation and when the *we-image* takes precedence over the *ego-image*, anything that happens to their country, the threat of war, an invasion or a serious economic or political crisis, immediately brings with it the fear of losing their own identity, of losing their own ego.

Even if someone feels oppressed, their resistance to react are paralysed by the identification with national values and ideals that could ensure not only the survival of the state but their own personal survival. In other words, the resistance of individuals is paralysed in the face of the forces of the oppressor. A total servitude to the national ideal and to the leaders of the nation in a quest for the protection of their oppressors. Norbert Elias thus explains the German people's *desire for submission*. An individual can free themselves from oppression by means of resistance and rebellion. However, the possibility of resisting is bound up with the separation between their own ideals and values and collective ideals and values, or to put it another way, when subjugated peoples are able to differentiate themselves from their oppressive rulers. "When their system of ideals and values is more or less identical with that of their masters", says Elias, "when their own conscience and we-ideal is on the side of the oppressors, the negative components of their feeling-set towards the oppressors cannot be directly and openly expressed" (Elias 1989: 379). In Ferenczi's words, we find an idea very close to that of Elias: "Now, in situations where protest and negative reaction, that is, all criticism and expression of discontent, are forbidden, criticism can find expression only in as indirected forma" (Ferenczi 1932b: 50). Traumatised individuals are silenced by the oppressor and remain incapable of articulating resistance or objections, or of expressing any opinion of their own.

Ferenczi furthermore states that in cases where protest or any criticism or expression of discontent are forbidden: "The annihilated part of the person falls into a state of decay and decomposes. Should the entire person be prevented from acting, then generalized decomposition ensues, that is to say, death" (Ferenczi 1932b: 88). But the fear of a violent death leads to a dissociation between feelings and thoughts. Actions are immobilized and conflicts are now reproduced in the psychic processes of the individual themselves. Norbert Elias writes,

> The tensions and conflicts between subjects and masters, oppressed and oppressors, become internal tensions and conflicts of the ruled and oppressed themselves. Hands which might otherwise be raised against the masters become paralysed. (...) The main battleground of the conflict shifts from the inter-human to the intra-human level.
>
> (Elias 1989: 379–380)

The intrapsychic conflict, expressed via the *lust for submission*, can take other directions. Instead of turning on the individual themselves, rendering them completely subjugated to the oppressor, it can take the form of outward aggression, in a *lust for aggression*. Norbert Elias continues as follows: "The hostility which is blocked from consciousness and expression in relation to powerful superiors may show itself as resentment or hatred against people who are, or appear to be, socially inferior and weaker" (Elias 1989: 380). This return of violence towards more vulnerable people, Elias writes, helps to understand the mechanisms that led the German people to seek to destroy the Jewish people. This is what Elias goes on to describe in the stance of cyclist, the *Radfahrer*, who bows his head to those who are in front and treads on those individuals who are beneath him.

To suggest a relationship between two authors who, as far as we know, had not close dealings with each other, is a challenge we acknowledge, as we recognize important changes in the way that Norbert Elias understands the dynamic of the civilizing process. Up to this point the civilizing process has shown how social structures are organized around the repression of urges, whose transference to the background of psychic life leads to thoughts, habits and emotions that establish hegemonic social classes and groups in search of privileges, power and exclusion. In this way, we can say that the exclusionary, colonizing dynamic of the civilizing process led to the expansionism of the great nation-states, to nationalist ideals, to religious intolerance, to belief in the superiority of certain races, as well as to the production of weapons of mass destruction that very nearly wiped out humanity in its entirety.

At the end of his work, Norbert Elias cannot fail to investigate the effects of the *decivilizing process* caused by the very highest societies. Based on his theory about decivilizing processes, we must also comprehend the mechanisms on which civilizations are constructed. Not only repression, but also denial. Not only acts of violence, but also traumas and catastrophes. The collapse of civilization, which resulted in the genocidal project to construct a new Reich, diverted the German civilizing process towards a *regression towards barbarism*, causing traumas, deaths and destruction. All this in the name of civilization.

References

Elias, Norbert (1939) *The Civilizing Process. Sociogenetic and Psychogenetic Investigations*, ed. by E. Dunning, J. Goudsblom and S. Mennell, trans. by E. Japhcott. Oxford: Blackwell Publishing, 2013.

——— (1989) *The Germans. Power Struggles and the Development of Habitus in the Nineteenth and Twentieth Centuries*, trans. by E. Dunning and S. Mennell. New York: Columbia University Press, 1996.

Elias, Norbert and Scotson, John L. (1965) *The Established and the Outsiders – A Sociological Enquiry into Community Problems*. London: Sage Publications, 1994.

Ferenczi, Sándor (1928) "The Adaptation of the Family to the Child", in *Final Contributions to the Problems and Methods of Psycho-analysis*, ed. by M. Balint, trans. by E. Mosbacher. London/New York: Routledge, 2018.

——— (1931) "The Child Analysis in the Analysis of Adults", in *Final Contributions to the Theory and Technique of Psycho-Analysis*, ed. by M. Balint, trans. by E. Mosbacher et al. London: Routledge, 2018.

——— (1932a) "Notes and Fragments", in *Final Contributions to the Theory and Technique of Psycho-Analysis*, ed. by M. Balint, trans. by E. Mosbacher et al. London: Routledge, 2018.

——— (1932b) *The Clinical Diary of Sándor Ferenczi*, ed. by J. Dupont, trans. by M. Balint and N. Jackson. Cambridge, MA/London: Harvard University Press, 1988.

——— (1933) "Confusion of Tongues between Adults and the Child", in *Final Contributions to the Theory and Technique of Psycho-Analysis*, ed. by M. Balint, trans. by E. Mosbacher et al. London: Routledge, 2018.

Foulkes, S. H. (1937) "On Introjection", in *Selected Papers. Psychoanalysis and Group Analysis*, ed. by E. Foulkes. London: Karnak Books, 1990.

Freud, Anna (1936) *The Ego and the Mechanisms of Defence*. London: Karnak Books, 1992.

Freud, Sigmund (1915) "Thought on the Times of War and Death", in *The Standard Edition of the Complete Psychological Work of Sigmund Freud – On the History of Psycho-Analytic Movement, Papers on Metapsychology and Other Works (1914–1916)*, vol. XIV, ed. and trans. by J. Strachey. London: Hogarth Press, 1981.

——— (1920) "Beyond the Pleasure Principle", in *The Standard Edition of the Psychoanalytical Works of Sigmund Freud: Beyond the Pleasure Principle, Group Psychology and Other Works (1920–1922)*, vol. XVIII, ed. and trans. by J. Strachey. London: Hogarth Press, 1981.

——— (1921) "Group Psychology and the Analysis of the Ego", in *The Standard Edition of the Complete Psychological Work of Sigmund Freud – Beyond the Pleasure Principle, Group Psychology and Other Works (1920–1922)*, vol. XVIII, ed. and trans. by J. Strachey. London: Hogarth Press, 1981.

——— (1926) "Inhibition, Symptoms and Anxiety", in *The Standard Edition of the Complete Psychological Works of Sigmund Freud: An Autobiographical Study, Inhibition, Symptoms and Anxiety, The Question of Lay Analysis and Other Works (1925–1926)*, vol. XX, ed. and trans. by J. Strachey. London: Hogarth Press, 1981.

——— (1927) "Fetishism", in *The Standard Edition of the Complete Psychological Works of Sigmund Freud – The Future of an Illusion, Civilization and its Discontents and Other Works (1927–1931)*, vol. XXI, ed. and trans. by J. Strachey. London: Hogarth Press, 1981.

——— (1933) "Why War", in *The Standard Edition of the Complete Work of Sigmund Freud – New Introductory Lectures on Psycho-analysis and Other Works (1932–1936)*, vol. XXII, ed. and trans. by J. Strachey. London: Hogarth Press, 1981.

——— (1939) "Moses and the Monotheism", in *The Standard Edition of the Complete Psychological Works of Sigmund Freud – Moses and Monotheism, an Outline of Psychoanalysis and Other Works (1937–1939)*, vol. XXIII, ed. and trans. by J. Strachey. London: Hogarth Press, 1981.

——— (1940) "Splitting of the Ego in the Process of Defence", in *The Standard Edition of the Complete Psychological Works of Sigmund Freud – Moses and Monotheism, An Outline of Psycho-analysis and Other Works (1937–1939)*, vol. XXIII, ed. and trans. by J. Strachey. London: Hogarth Press, 1981.

——— (2010) *Sigmund Freud – Unterdeß halten wir zusammen: Briefe an die Kinder*. Berlin: Aufbau Verlag.

Torok, Maria (2001) "Catastrophes [Katasztrófak] Lettre ouverte sur la correspondance de Freud avec Ferenczi", in *La psychanalyse avec Nicolas Abraham et Maria Torok*, ed. by Jean-Claude Rouchy. Toulouse: Érès, "Transition", p. 81–83. www.cairn.info/la-psychanalyse-avec-nicolas-abraham-et-maria-toro-9782865869152-page-81.htm

Tubert-Oklander, Juan (2019) "Ferenczi and Group Analysis", in *Psychoanalysis, Group Analysis and Beyond. Towards a New Paradigm of the Human Being*. London/New York: Routledge, 2022.

7 Freud's Moses

A historical novel

Despite the signs of the arrival of more sombre times, Sigmund Freud resisted leaving Vienna until the very last moment. Feeling protected within his country's borders, he did not believe that the mounting danger of neighbouring Germany would reach his home. In April 1933, three weeks after the *Reichstag* fire, he had stood firm in him position when answering a colleague and friend, the Hungarian psychoanalyst Sándor Ferenczi, who was already encouraging him to flee:

> I am not considering leaving Vienna. I am not mobile enough, too dependent on treatment, little alleviations and comforts, also don't like to leave my property in the lurch, but I would probably also remain if I were intact and youthfully fresh. An emotional attitude naturally lies at the base of this decision, but there is also no lack of rationalizations. It is not certain that the Hitler regime will also over power Austria; it is, of course, possible, but everyone believes that it will not reach the height of brutality here that it has in Germany. There is certainly no personal danger for me, and if you assume life in oppression to be amply uncomfortable for us Jews, then don't forget how little contentment life promises refugees in a foreign country, be it Switzerland or England. Flight, I think, would be justified only in the case of lethal danger, and incidentally, if they kill you, it's one kind of death like any other.
>
> (Freud 2000: 449)

But things rapidly got worse. On 12 March 1938, without the firing of a single shot and without encountering any political resistance, Nazi Germany annexed Austria as a province of the New Reich. That same day Freud wrote in his diary: "*Finis Austriæ*" (Freud 1992: 229). Three days later, an SA group broke into his home and on the 22nd of that month, his daughter Anna was taken by the Gestapo to give a statement about the suspicion that the *International Psychoanalytical Association* was a Zionist and anti-Nazi institution. Freud definitively left the home where he had lived for almost four decades on 4 June 1938, with swastika flags hanging from the windows in his building, number 19 Berggasse street. His notoriety and the influence of important friends helped him to secure permission from the Nazi

DOI: 10.4324/9781003378938-7

party to leave Vienna, although it also entailed the payment of a significant sum to the German government. With the assistance of his friend Ernest Jones, he settled in London at 20 Maresfield Gardens, accompanied by his wife Martha, daughter Anna and Paula Fichtl, their governess. Ernst Freud, their eldest son, awaited the arrival of his relatives in the English capital, where he had been living and working as an architect since 1933. Freud spent the last fifteen months of his life in London, where treated his last patients and wrote his last texts.

Written between 1934 and 1938, at a time when German students were burning books by Jewish authors in public squares, as happened in Berlin on 10 May 1933 on the initiative of Joseph Goebbels, Nazi minister of propaganda, *Moses and Monotheism* [*Der Mann Moses und die monotheistische Religion: Drei Abhandlungen*] explores the lead-up to the persecutions of the Jewish people, as Freud himself announced in a letter to Arnold Zweig, dated 30 September 1934: "Faced with the new persecutions, one asks oneself again how the Jews have come to be what they are and why they have attracted this undying hatred" (Freud 1970: 91). However, the issues dealt with in this work became more important than he had stated when they addressed the theme of intolerance towards the other as a universal of humanity itself. The Jewish question is presented to underline that the aim of psychoanalysis had always been to reveal the disquieting strangeness that characterizes the place of alterity, showing that identities simultaneously bear the marks of the familiar and the strange.

Freud, throughout his life, had always been a stranger wherever he went. A stranger in the domain of reason, for declaring that we are determined by unconscious processes. A stranger within medicine, for revealing that some of our symptoms are created by our brains. A stranger within Judaism, for proclaiming himself an atheist Jew. A stranger among his countrymen, for not recognising himself as Austrian. However, he was a stranger within psychoanalysis itself for searching for the bases of his ideas in literature, sociology, anthropology, philosophy, and mythology, always revisiting his theories as they developed from his clinical work.

The Germans by Norbert Elias (1989) and Sigmund Freud's *Moses and Monotheism* (1939) are both mature works, characterized by issues that led both authors to revisit their origins at the same time as reflecting on the discontent of their eras. Late works that converge and dialogue with each other, although they were published over 60 years apart. What invites us to compare these two ostensibly dissociated works, one of which discusses the origin of the Jewish people and the other that of the Germans, is the ways in which their authors think about the incidence of traumatic events as the link between the transformations in the social structure and the changes in psychological structures, as well as the effects of repression on the repetition of this trauma, no longer as a memory but as an act. Furthermore, a same understanding seems to underpin the two works, namely that our psychological structure is not isolated from social processes. These are two works in which their authors unearth from the lacunae and distortions of historical narratives what remained unsaid, whether because it was forgotten or because it was denied, and is passed on over the generations as traumatic events that are brought up to date whenever civilization is under threat.

7.1 The civilizing process of Jewish monotheism

The two introductory notes that Freud wrote for the text *Moses and Monotheism*, one in March 1938, a few months after being forced to leave Vienna, and the other in June 1938, just after his arrival in London, illustrate the passage of two points in time that contradict and even cancel each other out. In the interval between the one and the other, threats and intolerance were directed at the Freud family. Shortly before leaving his home, he recognized the danger that was on his doorstep, as he describes in the first introduction: "We are living in an especially remarkable period. We find to our astonishment that progress has allied itself with barbarism" (Freud 1939: 54). In Russia, where socialism was freeing the people from "opium" and the oppressions of the Church but was incarcerating freedom of thought in terms of political ideology, in Italy, where the growing wave of fascism led by Benito Mussolini, and in Germany, which was returning to barbarism under the guise of conservativism, everywhere there were movements to decivilize.

Influenced by the ideas he had written about in *The Future of an Illusion*, according to which religion serves to protect human beings from their state of helplessness and vulnerability, Freud still considered the Catholic Church as the last stronghold of protection. Consequently, he goes on to write in the first introduction of 1934: "The new enemy, to whom we want to avoid being of service, is more dangerous than the old one with whom we have already learnt to come to terms" (Freud 1939: 55). At that time, in his view it would have been preferable to live in the shadows of civilization, even if protected by an illusion than to live in total darkness. His fear, as he wrote a few years earlier in a letter to Arnold Zweig, was that his text about Moses would cause problems for his colleagues and also for the future of psychoanalysis in the world. In the end, without anyone foreseeing it, the dark times arrived and obliterated not only the freedom of individuals but the very human condition itself.

Thus, Freud succumbed to exile as the last alternative in order to survive. In the second preface to *Moses and Monotheism*, of 1938, he recognizes the following:

> At the earlier date I was living under the protection of the Catholic Church, and was afraid that the publication of my work would result in the loss of that protection and would conjure up a prohibition upon the work of the adherents and students psycho-analysis in Austria. Then, suddenly, came the German invasion and Catholicism proved, to use the words of the Bible, "a broken reed". In the certainty that I should now be persecuted not only form my line of thought but also for my "race" – accompanied by many of my friends, I left the city which, from early childhood, had been my home for seventy-eight years.
>
> (Freud 1939: 57)

Moses and Monotheism is a work that can be understood in multiple ways. Developed when old age no longer allowed Freud to take control of the direction of his own life and finished when exile seemed to be the only alternative to save his life. This text can be considered a last will and testament work by Freud, a text to pass on his ideas in response to all the opposition and resistance, including his own, to psychoanalysis and its institutions. It is a work that links together areas such as religion, anthropology, and the history of antiquity to show that civilization and barbarism come together via the insertion of the drive circuit in the political field. From the perspective of psychoanalysis, this work presents the problem of the relationship between social phenomena and the psychic economy in a more incisive way, considering the incidence of traumatic events in the imbrication between the individual and society.

In *Moses and Monotheism*, Freud returns to fundamental themes that he had developed a few years earlier. The myth of the murder of the father of the primitive horde and the formation of religion based on totemic societies, as explored in *Totem and Taboo*, of 1913, and the identificatory processes that connect individuals within communities, the basis of the ideas put forward in *Group Psychology and the Analysis of the Ego*, of 1921, are some of these premises that reappeared in this 1938 work, again linking social psychology to the psychology of the individual.

Nevertheless, if up to this point it was Freud who helped us to read Elias, how it was Elias who assisted us in reading Freud. Thus, it seems possible to see *Moses and Monotheism* as a work in which the Jewish people and their religion, viewed through their origins and their customs, can be read in the light of the theory of the civilizing process. From this perspective, the logic of the configuration involving established groups and outsiders helps us to see how certain character traits of the Jewish people were turned into a tradition for their descendants.

Unlike the mythical character who was passed on via holy scriptures, we can argue that Moses the man – and for this reason Freud entitled his text *Der Mann Moses* – is a construction that allows Freud to explore the civilizing process of the Jewish religion and the Jewish people. His reading of the origins of the Jewish religion operates in the same way as he used to investigate neurotic symptoms, revealing truths that were distorted in the formation process of *habitus* and the emotions of the Jewish people. The question of origins becomes the driving force behind this text that was one of Freud's last essays. From this starting point, his research expanded to unravel the destinies of civilization, to the place of the stranger, to intolerance of difference and to hatred of the other, positioning drive-based violence and decivilizing forces at the heart of civilizing processes.

The book *Moses and Monotheism* is made up of three chapters of different lengths that often repeat the main arguments as if they needed to emphasize plot how his theories – so full of questions – fit together. Despite having been written in 1934, the two first essays, "Moses an Egyptian" [*Moses ein Ägypter*] and "If Moses Was an Egyptian" [*Wenn Moses ein Ägypter war*], were published only in 1937, in the journal *Imago*. Together with the third essay, "Moses, His People, and Monotheistic Religion" [*Moses, sein Volk, und die Monotheistische Religion*], written in 1938, they make up the work, alongside two introductory notes, included at the start of the third essay, as well as what can be termed a third preface, situated halfway through the third essay, which summarizes and reiterates the theories that have been constructed up to that point. The publication of the work, its "like a bronze statue with feet of clay" (Freud 1939: 17), as Freud himself described it, only came about in 1939, during his exile in London.

Right in the first essay his investigations into the origin of the Jewish people again relate the topic of identity to psychoanalysis. Following the concept that the ego is a stranger to itself, Freud breaks with the notion of identity as a closed, substantial, and immutable structure, to state that, via identifications, the ego is established in an open, historical and procedural way. Individuals form their personalities through identificatory processes that involve not only individual ideals, in other words, who I admire or would like to be, but also social ideals. Different social configurations, like families, social classes, religious communities and even nation-states, in turn, are organized as social structures via the identificatory ties that individuals establish with each other.

In this way, Freud's criticisms of substantialist conceptualisations of identity link up with Elias's thinking when he proposes the concept of configuration to think about the network of interdependence between individuals, when he states that we cannot talk about *self-identity* without thinking about *we-identity* (Elias 1989) and when he develops the notion of *homines aperti* to differentiate from the closed structure of *homo clausus*. Both for the formation of the identities of individuals and for the formation of collective identities, what we find is a plurality of discourses always open to transformation.

As Freud returns to the relationship between changes in social structures and their effects on psychic structures, some of the theses developed in *Group Psychology and the Analysis of the Ego* reappear in *Moses and Monotheism* to describe the process of identification of each individual's *ego ideal* with the *we-ideal* of their group, represented, as we will see below, by the figure of the leader. However, the theses are not restricted to the process of establishing singular and collective identities. By illustrating the ambivalences of these processes, issues relating to xenophobia, social segregation, racism, and religious intolerance are put forward. Freud's research, in this sense, helps us to understand the hatred towards the Jewish people as an effect of a decivilizing process present in all relationships where an individual or a society's borders feel threatened. All the real and rational justifications to help explain this hostile emotion, however, are inadequate for the task, according to Freud. We need to go much deeper and describe the metapsychology of the civilizing process of Jewish monotheism.

In the same way as when he treated his patients, Freud constructs the *family novel* [*der Familienroman*] of the Jewish people based on the story of Moses, its founder. This phrase, which provides the title for a text published in 1909 and is part of the first proposed title of the work, *The Man Moses, a Historical Novel* [*Der Mann Moses, ein historischer Roman*], references the fantasies that reinvent the origins of children in other family ties, normally substituting the original parents for other more noble, wealthier ones. These are fantasies that unlock the child from the obligation to respond to paternal authority and inscribe conflicts between different generations as the basis of the progress of societies.

They are, however, nothing other than a process of working through the loss of a more satisfactory childhood past: "Indeed the whole effort at replacing the real father by a superior one is only an expression of the child's longing for the happy, vanished days when his father seemed to him the noblest and strongest of men and his mother the dearest and loveliest of women" (Freud 1909: 240–241), Freud states. Just as happens in individuals' histories, it is also possible to find in the histories of societies the construction of fantasies where ancestors are overrated. This is why questioning the truth of the story of the founder of the Jewish people was a personal heresy that Freud was committing against his own origins. "To deprive a people of the man whom they take pride in as the greatest of their sons" (Freud 1939: 7), he recognizes, was not an easy task. Even so, it cannot be abandoned for any reason. Not even national interests should be capable of interrupting the work of delving into the secrets of a people silently passed on in their traditions.

Let us then return to the text *Moses and Monotheism* to conduct a reading of Freud in the light of Norbert Elias's theory. Our understanding is that we can find in Freud's analyses of the formation of Jewish monotheism the directions taken by the civilizing process: the change in the balance of external coercions into self-coercions, the formation of behaviours and *habitus* that lead to a different, more stable self-control, as well as a rise in the level of mutual identification between individuals. Furthermore, in this re-reading using Elias's framework, the theory about the configuration between established groups and outsiders also helps us to understand the transformations of psychic structures in accordance with the changes in social structures.

In his first essay, "Moses an Egyptian", Freud begins from the hypothesis that the origins of Moses trace back to a foreigner: "Moses was an Egyptian – probably an aristocrat – whom the legend was designed to turn into a Jew" (Freud 1939: 15). Just as in the legends and myth that narrate the birth of heroes, the duplication of the origin of Moses was a way of guaranteeing the greatness and superiority of this great man, legislator and founder of the monotheist religion. In the case of the biblical story, however, there is an inversion of the narrative structure. In the Book of Exodus, we find the following: "When the child grew older, she brought him to Pharaoh's daughter, and he became her son. She named him Moses, 'Because', she said, 'I drew him out of the water'" (Exodus 2:10). Instead of describing what normally happens in stories that recount the birth of heroes, where the original family is of high nobility and the new adoptive family, poorer and more humble, in the biblical story of Moses, Freud says, the invented family is the one that abandoned him when he was a child and the Egyptian royal family, that saves him from the water, is his real family. A legend created by the Jewish people themselves as an attempt to wipe out the Egyptian origins of the leader of the Hebrews. A denial that eliminates the fundamental role of alterity in the constitutions of individuals and societies. A negation that ends up making the schisms in identity disappear and that creates resistance to any totalising idea.

Freud then begins to tell his story: it all began in the 18th dynasty of Egypt, in around 1375 BC, when a young pharaoh called Amenophis IV, assumed the throne and decided to ban polytheism and impose a new religion on Egyptians. A rigorous, universalized, and nationalized monotheism, that defended the absolute belief in a single divinity, Aten, the Sun God. This new religion, however, reached only part of the population, particularly those who made up the upper class of priests and the most dominant, spiritualized sector. The pharaoh also decided to change his name to Akhenaten, as a tribute to the new god, and to build a new royal residence. But this was not enough, and he demanded that his people believed exclusively in this single god, prohibiting and eradicating from temples all the inscriptions of the word "god" in the plural. For the first time in history, religious intolerance was established.

Since Akhenaten's monotheism had not been so popularized, remaining confined to a small circle of people around him, his legacy did not last for long. Straight after his death, seventeen years after his coronation, the new religion was eradicated from society, its temples were destroyed and the memory of the king was wiped out by some members of the oppressed clergy and the discontented majority of the population, who did not accept the sudden and violent imposition of a new religion. The fury and thirst for revenge led them to try to eliminate once and for all the memory of the heretic pharaoh. The golden age of the first experiment in monotheism immediately fell into oblivion. But forgetting history, as we know, is not synonymous with wiping it out or destroying it.

If until this point historiography has been able to prove facts, to argue that the bases of Jewish monotheism date back to Egyptian origins of the political and religious leader of the Hebrews, Freud had to make us of the construction of his hypothesis, the *historical novel* of the Jewish people: among those close to the pharaoh Akhenaten was Moses, a high-standing priest and passionate follower of the new religion of Aten. Following the rejection of Egyptian monotheism, Moses sought to keep alive his former leader's religion by founding a new empire. Consequently, Freud writes: "It remains possible that the religion which Moses gave to his Jewish people was nevertheless his own – that is *an* Egyptian religion, though not *the* Egyptian religion" (Freud 1939: 20). By means of ancient Semitic tribes who had established themselves in Egypt long ago, but were forgotten and living in poverty and isolation, Moses tried to make up for the losses suffered with the demise of Akhenaten's monotheism, choosing those foreigners as *his* people to whom he could pass on *his* ideals.

In fact, what Moses did was pass on values, customs and traditions imposed by the religion of the god Aten. He created laws and commandments and was probably more severe and ruthless than his former leader, demanding more sacrifices and more obligations than had been demanded of the Egyptian people. Freud thus concluded: "if Moses was an Egyptian and if he communicated his own religion to the Jews, it must have been Akhenaten's, the Aten religion" (Freud 1939: 24). In this way Moses, a foreigner, established at the heart of Judaism an equally foreign religion, Egyptian monotheism. However, Moses did not just pass on a religion to the Jews. He also passed on customs and ceremonies that came from the Egyptian tradition, such as circumcision, as well as prohibitions and restrictions that helped to define the Jewish people.

In order to pass the monotheistic religion of the pharaoh Akhenaten and establish a new empire, "an lead them to develop an independent and self-confident national existence in another country – which was what in fact happened" (Freud 1939: 27), Moses must have taken with him, when he fled Egypt, a considerable number of people belonging to his people, as well as people close to him, who occupied important positions like priests and scribes. In the same logic as the configuration of established groups and outsiders, Freud writes that, for Moses, the Jews who followed him beyond their country "were to serve him as a superior substitute for the Egyptians he had left behind" (Freud 1939: 30), and thus they could not be deemed any less than them in any aspect. The idea thus came about of a *holy nation*, not just to show their superiority in relation to other groups, but also to prohibit contact and association between their members and other individuals from outside.

The sacrifices and relinquishments that had to be made due to the demands and coercions of a god who revealed himself to be jealous, harsh, and cruel with his faithful also increased the value that Egyptians attributed to themselves. In exile, they sought to distinguish themselves from all the other peoples as a more powerful and more cohesive group, passing on habits, customs, and traditions wherever they went. However, those who came from Egypt, according to Freud, were no longer the same people who had followed Moses, but their descendants. They knew how to preserve the memory they had of Moses, organizing themselves into configurations marked by the veneration of the god Aten.

It was not in a short space of time, but over a long period, perhaps more than two or three generations, that a new religion was created. It was also not in Egypt, nor at the foot of Mount Sinai, but in Kadesh, an oasis full of springs and wells, located in the northwest of the Sinai Peninsula, where the encounter between the two groups led to the adoption of this new monotheism. It was there that the Egyptian descendants joined forces with Semitic tribes who worshipped the god Yahweh, a volcano god, a bloodthirsty sinister demon, who wandered around at night and feared the light of day. About them "It is not even certain that his religion was a genuine monotheism, that it denied the divinity of the deities of other peoples" (Freud 1939: 50), Freud writes. Further on he concludes that "the god Yahweh certainly bore no resemblance to the Mosaic god" (Freud 1939: 63).

In comparison to the Semitic tribes, the Egyptians formed a more cohesive group, whose individual members identified much more with each other through a leader, at the same time as being subjected to obligations, customs and ceremonies imposed by the monotheist religion. They brought with them more stable traditions, something which the others lacked. According to Freud: "The former Egyptians were probably fewer in numbers than the others, but showed themselves culturally the stronger" (Freud 1939: 38). Composing a more established group, the Egyptian descendants managed to ensure that the idea of absolute, universal and intolerant monotheism, one that was heavy on ceremonies and sacrifices, prevailed over Semitic tribes that, much more dispersed and fragmented, worshipped the god Yahweh with denying the existence of the gods of the other tribes. Yahweh thus gradually lost his characteristics and took on those that characterized the identity of Aten, Moses's former god.

The relationship between the established group and the outsider groups helps us to understand not only the nature of the Jewish people, but also the hatred that other peoples directed at them. According to Freud these were motives that can only be found in the unconscious determinations of the civilizing process of this people. Freud writes:

> We may start from a character-trait of the Jews which dominates their relation to others. There is no doubt that they have a particularly high opinion of themselves, that they regard themselves as more distinguished, of a higher stranding, as superior to other people – from whom they are also distinguished by many of their customs. At the same time they are inspired by a peculiar confidence in life, such as is derived from the secret ownership of some precious possession, a kind of optimism: pious people would call it trust in God.
>
> (Freud 1939: 105)

The pride and self-confidence of the Jews was probably passed on by Moses through the belief that they had been chosen as God's people and that they were thus closer to Him. The Jewish people therefore not only distinguished themselves as superior and more powerful beings but excluded all others who were not recognized as similar to them. Freud continues: "He [Moses] raised their self-esteem by assuring them that they were the God's chosen people, he enjoined them to holiness and pledged them to be apart from others" (Freud 1939: 106). Within the relationship between established and outsider groups, barriers are created that prohibit the established from coexisting or having contact with members of the marginalized group. In the event of such contact occurring, the individual in question becomes a taboo in the eyes of his own group, a threat to the integrity and the cohesion of the most powerful.

To answer the question how it is possible that one man alone can demonstrate his efficiency in such an extraordinary way, Freud turns to an analysis of the relationship of the Jews with Moses, the great man [*der grosse Mann*], returning to the theses developed in *Group Psychology and the Analysis of the Ego*. In this text of 1921, the figure of the leader appears in the place of the *we-ideal* of each group, formed by identificatory processes between each individual's *ego-ideals*. A configuration that organizes itself through a leader, whether a person, an idea or even an emotion: "*A primary group of this kind is a number of individuals who have substituted one and the same object for their ego ideal and have consequently identified themselves with one another in their ego*", says Freud (Freud 1921: 116). Groups are constituted via emotional ties between their members and between individuals and a leader.

At the base of these identificatory processes are narcissistic structures that include those who are identical and exclude those who are different. In other words, an individual incorporates in the form of the ego ideal, the qualities of the individual or group with which they identify as if those qualities were their own. In this way, identifications are constantly transforming the structures of personality. In the formation of configurations, then, what we find are numerous egos collectivized by the process of mutual identification with a common *we-ideal.*

Individuals belonging to any type of social configuration feel loved and recognized by the leader, the representative of the *we-ideal*, to the same degree as they submit and sacrifice themselves to the leader's demands. The leader, in turn, occupies the place of someone who stands out from the members of the group, but also needs the group to exist. A configuration that organizes itself through relationships of interdependence. In the same way that parents need children in order to occupy a place of authority, or a king needs courtiers to maintain a position of power, the control and dominance that the leader exerts over his followers reflects his need to be loved and valued, just like Moses needed his entourage of Egyptian followers to pass on his religion via the establishment of a new empire.

This brings us back to the text *Moses and Monotheism* and the view that Moses, by occupying the position of leader, represents the *we-ideal* to the Jews. An authority that Jews identify with and that influences them not only through his personality, his actions, and his spiritual qualities, but also because of his ideas. As we have seen, Freudian theory shows that for both the psychology of groups and the psychology of individuals, the authorities emerge out of the necessity for love and protection on the part of members of the group. By establishing unconditional monotheism, Moses passed on to the Jewish people a relationship of dependence with an authority that brings together, around this figure, identificatory ties between the members of a community as if they were children belonging to the same family. Identificatory processes thus transfer to the political sphere the same emotions, contradictory and ambivalent as they always are, that circulate in the most intimate, family relationships. Freud therefore succeeds in approximating the authority of Moses with paternal authority:

> There is no doubt that it was a mighty prototype of a father which, in the person of Moses, stooped to the poor Jewish bondsmen to assure them that they were his dear children. And no less overwhelming must have been the effect upon them of the idea of an only, eternal, almighty God, to whom they were not too men for him to make a covenant with them and who promised to care for them if they remained loyal to his worship.
>
> (Freud 1939: 110)

According to Freud, individuals link up with each other, recognising themselves as legitimate members of the same group, through identification with the leader. The sense of belonging to a group with high social value gives individuals narcissistic satisfaction, at the point when the ego ideals and the *we-ideals* are one and the same. In this way they manage to feel loved and protected. A love that, to be given, demands as payment submission and sacrifice. They consequently avoid the *anxiety* [*soziale Angst*] created by the threat of exclusion or of breaking emotional ties between members of the group.

According to Freud's hypotheses, the nature of the Jewish people was created through processes of identification with Moses, who gave Jews the idea of a single great, almighty god. "Anyone who believed in this God had some kind of share in his greatness, might feel exalted himself" (Freud 1939: 112), Freud writes. This group's *we-ideals*, when identified with the ego ideal of each individual, imprinted the mark of superiority, passed on by Moses as an attribute of God himself. It was a way of being able to share in God's greatness, at the same time as excluding the possibility of contact and coming together with other groups. A sentiment that can be likened to the pride in belonging to a powerful nation and that cannot be found among citizens of states whose sovereignty is constantly threatened or subjugated by other states. To quote Freud:

> Thus, pride in the greatness of the British Empire has a root as well in the consciousness of the greater security – the protection – enjoyed by the individual Briton. This may resemble the conception of a grand God. And, since one can scarcely claim to assist God in the administration of the world, the pride in God's greatness fuses with the pride of being chosen by him.
>
> (Freud 1939: 112)

Moses, the supreme authority of the Jewish people, imposes on his subjects unconditional obedience to a series of coercions, ceremonies and habits that must be reproduced as an unbreakable tradition to avoid the risk of not being recognized as similar to other members of the community or even being expelled from it: "One must admire him, one may trust him, but one cannot avoid being afraid of him too" (Freud 1939: 110). As well as the belief of having been chosen by God as a superior people and sharing in His greatness, spiritual development and the subsequent renunciation of impulses, constitute the civilizing process of Jewish monotheism.

Prohibiting the creation of images of God, following the model imposed by Akhenaten in the religion of the god Aten, is a renunciation that implies a profound transformation in the psychic economy. Like the power of a repression, this prohibition imposes the abandonment of sensory perceptions in favour of abstract representations. A cultural development in which spirituality triumphs over sensibility, in a series of transformations that gradually shape the nature of the Jewish people. As an effect of this civilizing process, habits are instilled as a way of attributing to oneself superior values of power and prestige that at the same time reproduce logics of exclusion and segregation.

Circumcision was one of these customs that, over the centuries, saw its meaning become distorted. It is a "key-fossil", as Freud came to see it, as it becomes a vestige that is historically preserved. Via circumcision it is possible to reconstruct certain events forgotten as a result of the civilizing process of the Jewish people. Passed on by Moses to his followers as a legacy of a popular Egyptian practice, its objective was to establish identifications with ancestors at the same time as differentiating them from all other people who were not part of this community. In other words, by being a tradition, circumcision follow the totemic logic of aggrandisement of the group that practices it and marginalization of all those who do not share the same values. Circumcision becomes a tradition that confirms, every time it is put into practice, the established group status of the Jewish people. This custom, according to Freud:

> Those who do not practice it look on it as very strange and are a little horrified by it, but those who have adopted circumcision are proud of it. They feel exalted by it, ennobled, as it were, and look down with contempt on the others, whom they regard as unclean.
>
> (Freud 1939: 29–30)

As we know, transformations in social structures lead to profound changes in the psychic economy and dynamics of individuals. By instilling habits, customs and traditions, the development of spirituality gradually imposed on the Jewish people what Freud termed "renunciation of drives" [*Der Triebverzicht*]. It is not obvious, he says, that distancing sensuality from spirituality causes an increase in a person's or a people's self-confidence. The purpose is thus focused on seeking a meta-psychological understanding of this mechanism, so as to describe the control of drives that underlies the civilizing process of the Jewish people.

According to Freud, there are barriers in the external world that prevent the immediate satisfaction of drives, as well as barriers within individuals themselves, that prevent satisfaction being obtained. It may be that the ego avoids seeking satisfaction when it feels that this would put it in a position of danger, for example. This is what Freud called the reality principle. In such cases, the ego renounces drive satisfaction and looks for other means of satisfaction that do not involve a direct encounter with the object of pleasure. However, drives may also be renounced for reasons inherent to psychic structures. Freud writes,

> In the course of an individual's development a portion of the inhibiting forces in the external world are internalized and an agency is constructed in the ego which confronts the rest of the ego in an observing, criticizing and prohibiting sense. We call this new agency the *super-ego*.
>
> (Freud 1939: 116)

Consequently, as well as the prohibitions that stem from the external world, the ego also must consider the impediments of the "internal world", in other words, the coercions of the superego itself.

With the development of large configurations like modern states, that have rendered more complex networks of interdependence and have increased the scope of identification, renouncing the satisfaction of drives has established more peaceful ways of coexisting in society. However, the conflicts that resulted from the external world's prohibitions have not been entirely eliminated but transferred to the background of the psyche. Norbert Elias thus returns to the psychoanalytical concept of the superego to illustrate the result of a process of internalization of external social coercions into self-coercions. This is an open, historical, and procedural psychic structure, in constant transformation whenever individuals establish new ties between each other. By means of identificatory processes, individuals gradually internalize as their own (*ego-ideals*) collective ideals (*we-ideals*) that they come across in groups, families, societies, religious communities, the state, in short, in the different social configurations that they form part of during their lives.

Contrary to what we might think, the functions of the superego are not restricted to the unconscious representation of social coercions. They also impose narcissistic ideals on the ego that serve drive needs. Thus, when Freud says that the demands of the superego lead to displeasure, but also to a significant economic gain in terms of satisfaction, what he is stating is that the pleasure gained results from when the ego agrees with the values and norms transmitted by this internalized authority figure. In these situations, "the ego feels elevated; it is proud of the instinctual renunciation, as though it were a valuable achievement" (Freud 1939: 117), Freud writes.

In periods of time when individuals were subjugated by external authorities, they felt protected and loved only when they obeyed the coercions imposed from the outside to counter their drive needs. The rest of the time, they lived in constant danger, at the mercy of threats that could come from anywhere. As an effect of the civilizing process, the ego seeks within the superego the equivalent of the protection and love that it received from the external authority that it was once dependent on. Consequently, Freud writes,

> the ego is apprehensive about risking the love of its supreme master; it feels his approval as liberation and satisfaction and his reproaches as pangs of conscience. When the ego has brought the super-ego the sacrifice of an instinctual renunciation, it expects to be rewarded by receiving more love from it. The consciousness of deserving this love is felt by it as pride.
>
> (Freud 1939: 117)

The renunciation of drives demanded by the civilizing process of Jewish monotheism, established by Moses, the great man, leader and legislator, gave Jews greater self-confidence via spiritual advancements. Freud thus drew an equivalence between this religious authority, the father and the superego. In all three cases what was passed on was the idea of a spiritual, ethical and intellectually superior figure, to whom everybody should submit, obeying his coercions and renouncing the satisfaction of their drives. The power of renouncing drives made it possible to organise a social configuration characterized by identification between its members, at the same time as the exclusion of all those not subjected to the same commandments and prohibitions.

7.2 Transmission of civilization

In *Moses and Monotheism*, Freud brings the psychology of society and that of the individual into closer proximity, beginning with and expanding on the hypotheses put forward a few years earlier in *Totem and Taboo*. It was in this 1913 text that he first formulated a theory about how individuals established ties between each other, organizing themselves into the most different types of social configurations.

In this text we also find his elaborations on the transmission process of civilization in human communities over long periods of time. Freud writes: "This gives rise to two further questions: how much can we attribute to psychical continuity in the sequence of generations? And what are the ways and means employed by one generation in order to hand on its mental states to the next one?" (Freud 1913: 158). His conclusions, however, only proposed a single hypothesis about heredity, as he himself explains in the quote that follows: "A part of a problem seems to be met by the inheritance of psychical dispositions which, however, need to be given some sort of impetus in the life of the individual before they can be roused into actual operation" (Freud 1913: 158).

The Freudian theory of hereditary transmission appears to take a conservative, repetitive position that deems impossible changes in psychic structures in accordance with social transformations. In this sense, Stephen Frosh reaches the conclusion that in *Totem and Taboo*, "the past lives on unchanged, in the species as in the individual", such that "because of the nature of the instincts, certain scenarios will always be replayed, with a universal, repressive result" (Frosh 1987: 45). A universality that establishes individuals closed to their times and their society. However, Freud also recognizes the following: "If so, however, we may safely assume that no generation is able to conceal any of its more important mental processes from its successor" (Freud 1913: 159). Collective memories can never be erased or destroyed, even if they fall into oblivion, remaining alive and active in the unconscious.

In 1913 Freud established the bases of our societies from two elements, found in so-called "primitive" societies, i.e., societies most distanced from what is considered the height of civilization of contemporary European societies. On the one hand, *taboos* are defined as prohibitions and restrictions that, over a very long period of time, have been passed on and reproduced without individuals knowing their origins or intentions. Taboos served to regulate habits and customs, preventing certain drives from being acted on at the heart of human communities. As a characteristic of their structure, taboos contain an ambiguous mix of the sacred and the dangerous, being both prohibited and desired at one and the same time. In Freud's words,

> What we are concerned with, then, is a number of prohibitions to which these primitive races are subjected. Every sort of thing is forbidden; but they have no idea why, and it does not occur to them to raise the question. On the contrary, they submit to the prohibitions as though they were a matter of course and feel convinced that any violation of them will be automatically met by the direst punishment.
>
> (Freud 1913: 21)

Nevertheless, the origins of taboos are connected to the formation of another element, a force of authority, incontestable, endowed with powers and values that demand obedience and respect. These are *totems*, according to Freud, the foundation of the identities of all "primitive" communities. He continues:

> What is a totem? It is as a rule an animal (whether edible and harmless or dangerous and feared) and more rarely a plant or a natural phenomenon (such as rain or water), which stands in a peculiar relation to the whole clan.
>
> (Freud 1913: 2)

The members of a totemic clan believe they descend from the totem and expect to be protected and cared for by it. The totem is the common feature that transforms a multiplicity of individuals into a community, designating its *we-identity*. However, by establishing kinship relationships it also creates logics of exclusion. Exogamy and the horror of incest, as Freud writes in *Totem and Taboo*, are prohibitions that prevent certain relationships between members of the same totemic clan, for example.

In Freud's view, civilization is passed on via processes of identification and social coercions, the origins of which cannot be remembered by those who reproduce them, insofar as repression distorts their original meanings. Identification with totems and obedience to taboos lead to the repetition of patterns of behaviour that are founded on forgetting their origins and intentions, without being able to question or discuss them and only being able to respect and reproduce them. In this way it can be said that the origins of totem and taboos are unknown and incomprehensible, just like the origins of our habits and our customs are today for us. A naturalization that makes it impossible for anyone who reproduces them without knowing why to question them. However, in order for unconscious content to be passed on, Freud seems to need more explanations than those offered by his hereditary hypothesis.

In the text *The Ego and the Id*, of 1923, the question of the transmission of civilization is picked up again precisely in the chapter that deals with the origin of the superego and the ego ideal. It is no coincidence that Norbert Elias returned to this Freudian concept to formulate his theory about the civilizing process. In Freud's view, based on the remodelling of psychic structures and the consequent elaboration of the superego, it is no longer possible to say that patterns of behaviour are reproduced over generations either via heredity or via the power of consciousness. "Nevertheless it is not possible to speak of direct inheritance in the ego" (Freud 1923: 38), Freud writes, continuing as follows: "Moreover, one must not take the difference between ego and id in too hard-and-fast a sense, nor forget that the ego is a specially differentiated part of the id" (Freud 1923: 38). The transmission of repressed memories, that pass from generation to generation and are often perpetuated for many centuries, can only occur via unconscious processes.

Sigmund Freud and Norbert Elias, each in their own way, showed that the civilizing process can pass on content that, via the power of repression, is etched into the unconscious like a scar. Memories of experiences that cannot be erased or destroyed. Here is what Freud writes in his 1923 text about the processes by which civilization is passed on:

> The experiences of the ego seem at first to be lost for inheritance; but, when they have been repeated often enough and with sufficient strength in many individuals in successive generations, they transform themselves, so to say,

> into experiences of the id, the impressions of which are preserved by heredity. Thus is the id, which is capable of being inherited, are harboured residues of the existences of countless egos; and, when the ego forms it super-ego out of the id, it may perhaps only be reviving shapes of former egos and be bringing them to resurrection.
>
> (Freud 1923: 38)

Certain experiences are able to transform psychic structures when they are repeated with a degree of *repetition* and *strength*, in other words, over a long period of time and with intensity. Here, Norbert Elias helps us to reread Freud by viewing the historical and social aspects of the civilizing process into a long-term perspective. This sociologist already stated that experiences that are frequently and forcefully repeated over a long period of time, over generations or even centuries, manifest themselves as habits, customs, and traditions. These repetitive behaviours establish identities that situate individuals as members of the same configuration at the same time as excluding all those who are considered different. Gradually they are internalized and consequently create permanent marks on the id. Thus, the ego and the superego, by being formed from the Id, end up receiving and reproducing the same hegemonic patterns of behaviour that were unconsciously passed on from one generation to another.

What previously occurred externally in social relations is transferred to the background of the psyche and, in this way, is reproduced without individuals knowing why. Habits, customs, and traditions become formations of the unconscious in the same way that dreams, symptoms, and Freudian slips are described by Freud was individual formations. An important difference between them appears to be that the former, unlike symptoms, can collectivise individuals within social configurations via identificatory processes.

By extending the theory of the unconscious to the formation of social structures, Freud illustrates that the civilizing process is also marked by a series of traumas, ruptures and discontinuities caused by events that individuals and societies prefer not to know about. In one of his last texts, he strives to answer the questions that had been formulated in *Totem and Taboo* about the transmission of civilization throughout the generations. How does repressed content, that has been pushed into the background of the psyche and the obscure realms of societies, become cultural heritage? How does it cease to be part of the past and determine the life and future of a community? Freud's theory, outlined in this 1939 text, is based on the following argument. He states:

> What is forgotten is not extinguished but only "repressed"; its memory-traces are present in all their freshness, but isolated by "anticathexes". They cannot enter into communication with other intellectual processes; they are unconscious – inaccessible to consciousness.
>
> (Freud 1939: 94)

This point seems to be more obvious in the case of individual psychic processes than that of social structures. In the process of the constitution of the psyche, certain experiences are repressed and transferred to the unconscious, where they remain as content inaccessible to consciousness. In Freud's opinion, these untranslatable traces are not restricted to the traumatic experiences of individuals. If that were the case, we could not really talk about the transmission of civilization between different generations since the unconscious material would be revised in line with the particular experience of each individual. But that is not what Freud believed. In his view, social formations also preserve unconscious mnemonic traces. To quote Freud:

> But a fresh complication arises when we become aware of the probability that what may be operative in an individual's psychical life may include not only what he has experienced himself but also things that were innately present in him at his birth, elements with a phylogenetic origin – an *archaic heritage*. The questions then arise of what this consists in, what it contains and what is the evidence for it.
>
> (Freud 1939: 98)

What Freud refers to here as *archaic heritage* and what, in *Totem and Taboo*, corresponds to the hereditary transmission of constitutional elements, are "memory-trees of the experience of earlier generations" (Freud 1939: 99) that, at a given moment, ended up being forgotten. However, for Freud, nor Elias, was this about essentialist knowledge. Neither is it invariable, fixed, or permanent. Such knowledge is modified over time in accordance with social changes.

Thus, the description of the process of transmission of unconscious content from one generation to another becomes one of the most fundamental problems for psychoanalysis. Freud writes: "If we assume the survival of these memory-traces in the archaic heritage, we have bridged the gulf between individual and group psychology: we can deal with peoples as we do with an individual neurotic" (Freud 1939: 100). Freud therefore returns to his theories about the formation and transmission of content between psychic structures, as he had formulated in *The Ego and the Id*, where he describes how certain patterns of behaviour, that were repeated in the ego with *repetition* e *strength*, are gradually incorporated by the id and transformed into psychic dispositions that tend to be repeated.

In *Moses and Monotheism*, Freud responds to the question about the conditions in which an experience is transformed into an archaic heritage in the following way: "if the event was important enough, or repeated often enough, or both" (Freud 1939: 101), it is incorporated by the id. The unconscious incorporates the social changes of content whose *importance* and *frequency* stretches over a long period of time. Therefore, this material that has become unconscious begins to compulsively insist on being repeated. Called upon, so to speak, by present-day situations, it is driven to resurface, even in distorted form. Freud writes, "if at any time in recent experience impressions or experiences occur which resemble the repressed so closely that they are able to awaken it" (Freud 1939: 95). The forgotten mnemonic trace is re-awakened in the present day, revealing a truth that must be deciphered beyond the obvious events.

It is a question of ancestral knowledge, whose original meaning has been lost and needs to be deciphered so that its origins and purpose can be discovered. This concept is similar to Norbert Elias's idea of *second nature*, acquired from the internalization of behaviours, customs and social rules throughout the civilizing process.

7.3 Historical truth

As we know, Freud never went back on his ideas, even when he had to face up to the greatest resistance against psychoanalysis: "But apart from this we shall venture to maintain independence of the authorities and to 'proceed along our own track'" (Freud 1939: 37), he writes. Let us therefore follow the construction of his theories. In his opinion, Jewish monotheism originated from the principles of the Mosaic religion in Egypt, but only received due attention after a long period of time, that may have spanned two or three generations, until it was definitively established in Kadesh. A hiatus known as the *period of latency*, normally in reference to the formation process of psychic structures, but found in cases that involve traumatic events and, as we can see in *Moses and the Monotheism*, also in the formation processed of social structures. In all these situations, during this period, lacunae of memory are caused by negations *[Verneinung]* and denials *[Verleugnung]*, that distort *[Entstellung]* the linear linking together of histories.

Freud does not think it possible that the Egyptian Moses, who fled with the Jews from the persecutions of the pharaoh, had in fact been the same Moses of Kadesh, who established the new Jewish religion. When the two groups who came to form the new religion encountered each other, the descendants of those who were in Egypt would not renounce their memories of the liberation of their ancestors under the command of their leader. Still being very connected to the image of that great man, they wanted to keep his memory alive. For the others, in turn, it was important to state their devotion to the god Yahweh. Freud therefore concluded

> We are, I think, justified in separating the two figures and in assuming that the Egyptian Moses was never at Kadesh and had never heard the name of Yahweh, and that the Midianite Moses had never been in Egypt and knew nothing of Aten. In order to solder the two figures together, tradition or legend had the task of bringing the Egyptian Moses to Midian, and we have seen that more than one explanation of this was current.
>
> (Freud 1939: 41)

Once again, we see here both narratives about the birth of heroes, defining their identity via their relationship with the other. Two founders, two monotheisms, two gods, Aten and Yahweh. Gradually, the Egyptian Moses was being replaced by the Moses of Kadesh, transformed into a heroic, powerful and grandiose character. Two people condensed into the same figure. The Mosaic god was consequently not entirely forgotten, nor did he completely disappear from the memory of his people. A kind of memory of the god of Moses was preserved in a hidden form, like something *unspoken*, remaining active in the present time. As a result, the god Yahweh of the ancient tribes gradually acquired characteristics of the god of Moses's religion. He became hard and tough, a universal, brutalized god who reigns over everything and everybody. Yahweh was credited with having liberated the Jewish people. The shadow of the god that he had replaced, according to Freud, ended up becoming stronger than him. Freud writes,

> The religion of Moses, however, had not disappeared without leaving a trace. A kind of memory of it had survived, obscured and distorted, supported, perhaps, among individual members of the priestly caste by ancient records. And it was this tradition of a great past which continued to work in the background, as it were, which gradually gained more and more power over men's minds, and which finally succeeded in transforming the god Yahweh into the god of Moses and in calling back to life the religion of Moses which had been established and then abandoned long centuries earlier.
>
> (Freud 1939: 124)

The duality inherent in the origins of the Jewish religion retrace the interior alterity that set the bases of Egyptian monotheism in the figure of Moses, a foreigner who had to go into exile to establish a new people. In *Moses and Monotheism*, Freud condenses the formation process of neuroses as follows: "Early trauma – defence – latency – outbreak of neurotic illness – partial return of the repressed" (Freud 1939: 80). A formula that identifies the times when civilisation is passed on until a tradition is formed. By recognizing in social structures, the same process that occurs in the structure of individuals – as we see in the following quotation: "The reader is now invited to take the step of supposing that something occurred in the life of the human species similar to what occurs in the life of individuals" (Freud 1939: 80) –, Freud ends up expanding the concept of trauma. In the lives of both individuals and in societies there are events, many of which we do not even wish to know about, that leave permanent marks.

It is important to underline that the extent of the traumatic event does not necessarily reflect the occurrence of a single unexpected, violent event of great magnitude. According to Freud, all that is required is the existence of a *complemental series* of experiences, each of which alone could not lead to any trauma, but which end up combining their effects either through their importance, or their repetition, or both. A series of small shocks can be enough to leave its mark on the history of societies and of individuals in a traumatic way, when they occur with repetition and strength over a long period.

A long period of colonization or a socio-economic system based on slavery are collective traumatising experiences that can lead, as is the case in psychological traumas, to their *fixation* in a particular process and to *repetition compulsion*, in other words, the tendency to repeat and reproduce a traumatic event in the present time. In the same way, a state whose democratic regimes have been interrupted, resulting in the suspension of political freedom and constitutional rights, can easily reproduce the violence and oppression of those traumatic times if it does not know how to handle this past via reparation policies that seek to bring about justice for those who were directly and indirectly affected and to punish the perpetrators of that violence. The silencing of these traumas leads to fixations in these historical periods and consequently to their repetition, with them often appearing in a distorted way in other social configurations.

The traumatic survives in the web of social relationships like a foreign body that forces a society to reproduce the same suffering countless times throughout its history. This is the case of the maintenance of a different, divergent norm, "a State within a State" (Freud 1939: 76), in Freud's words, that forces the normal structure to act in a pathological way, repeating the "inner" suffering regardless of any "external" reality. This results in a rupture that preserves fragments of a memory but preventing it from being pieced together with the passage of time, in the same way that Freud described for his friend Wilhelm Fliess, in "Letter 52", regarding the inscription of psychic content. Freud writes,

> As you know, I am working on the assumption that our psychic mechanism has come into being by a process of stratification: the material present in the form of memory traces being subjected from time to time to a *rearrangement* in accordance with fresh circumstances – to a *retranscription*. Thus what is essentially new about my theory is the thesis that memory is present not once but several times over, that it is laid down in various kinds of indications.
>
> (Freud 1986: 207)

At that time, Freud described the psychic apparatus as a stratified memory system the contents of which, from time to time, are re-arranged and re-transcribed. Between one memory layer and another there must be a translation of psychic material. However, during this process, some errors can occur: "I explain the peculiarities of the psychoneuroses by supposing that this translation has not taken place in the case of some of the material, which has certain consequences" (Freud 1986: 208), Freud states. From the start of his clinical research, Freud recognized that content of a sexual nature, due to its powerful emotional charge, is difficult to work through in the transition between psychic phases. Excessive excitement provoked by a memory can reproduce the same intensity as the original event itself. Freud writes: "Thus, a sexual event in one phase acts in the next phase as though it were a current one and is accordingly uninhibitable" (Freud 1986: 209). But this is not only the case with regard to sexuality. As discussed above, events of a traumatic nature, like shocks, accidents or catastrophes, lead to an excess of excitement that resists being worked through. Therefore, a trauma always leads back to the same scene, tying the individual to the present time, as though the trauma can never stop happening.

Shifting away from what is proposed in the methodology adopted by Norbert Elias, who constructs his interpretation about the transformations in social structures from a long-term perspective, Freud condenses his narrative into a mythical construction. This does not mean, however, that he is denying the importance of the duration of social processes, much less inscribing a single, universal origin for all societies. Far from it. The story of the myth of the primitive horde, presented for the first time in *Totem and Taboo* and then returned to in *Moses and Monotheism*, is a condensed narrative that presents a logic of historical events that has repeated itself many times, with *repetition* and *strength*, over a long period of time. Freud writes, in a sentence that I would like to emphasize: "The story is told in an enormously condensed form, as though it had happened on a single occasion, while in fact it covered thousands of years and was repeated countless times during that long period" (Freud 1939: 81). An important history that has occurred time and again, over a long period and with great intensity, can be condensed into a single narrative, adopting the methodology that Freud proposed with his *construction in analysis*, without ignoring long-standing historical and social processes.

Freud thus returns to the myth presented in his book *Totem and Taboo*:

> The strong male was lord and father of the entire horde and unrestricted in his power, which he exercized with violence, All the females were his property wives and daughters of his own horde and some, perhaps, robbed from other hordes. The lot of his sons was a hard one: if they roused their father's jealousy they were killed or castrated or driven out, Their only resource was to collect together in small communities, to get themselves wives by robbery, and, when one or other of them could succeed in it, to raise them- 'selves into a position similar to their father's in the primal horde. For natural reasons, youngest sons occupied an exceptional position. They were protected by their mother's love, and were able to take advantage of their father's increasing age and succeed him on his death.
>
> (Freud 1939: 81)

A social configuration marked by primitivisms, animalities and ancestralities, in which every individual occupies a position of sovereign power over all others, monopolising not only physical violence but also the satisfaction of desires. The father of the horde was not subjected to any law, any coercion, or any restriction. All his sons, in turn, subjects of this absolutist sovereign, owed him unlimited obedience or risked being expelled from the group or even killed by him. Freud continues,

> The first decisive step towards a change in this sort of "social" organization seems to have been that the expelled brothers, living in a community, united to overpower their father and, as was the custom in those days, devoured him raw. There is no need to balk at this cannibalism; it continued far into later times.
>
> (Freud 1939: 81)

This Freudian construction serves as an analogy that condenses events that have occurred repeatedly throughout the course of history. At the individual level, the sons love and identify with their father, worshipping him as a role model at the same time as fearing his power. Paternal authority, that initially presents itself as external coercion, is gradually incorporated by the children as internal authority in the form of self-regulating structures. In this way, the functions of the superego reproduce in individuals the same structure of totemic societies, passing on not only prohibitions, via commandments such as "you cannot act like that", but also establishing identities and ideals, via declarations like "you should be like this". Following the killing of the father of the primate horde,

> The first form of a social organization came about with a *renunciation of instinct*, a recognition of mutual *obligations*, the introduction of definite institutions, pronounced inviolable (holy) – that is to say, the beginnings of morality and justice. Each individual renounced his ideal of acquiring his father's position for himself and of possessing his mother and sisters.
>
> (Freud 1939: 82)

At the level of social structures, individuals organize themselves in social configurations that regulate their drives through the establishment of rules and laws common to all. This was the case, for example, in court societies, as Elias describes in *The Civilizing Process*. Courtiers knew that they must guarantee their existence by submitting to customs and ceremonies that required them to control their drives. In this case, however, the king held the position of absolute authority, although he was still dependent on the rules of etiquette. Gradually, with the formation of modern states, individuals have come to recognize themselves as members of the same nation, without any of them having the right to occupy the position of sovereign.

Let us return to Freud's interpretation that the fate of Moses was wiped from history, in the same way as a murderer tries to rid himself of evidence of his crime. Freud writes: "In its implication the distortion of a text resembles a murder: the difficulty is not in perpetrating the deed, but in getting rid of its traces" (Freud 1939: 43). According to Freud, the exodus led by Moses occurred just after the end of the 18th Egyptian dynasty, with the death of Akhenaten between 1358 and 1350 B.C. Between the exile from Egypt and the taking of the holy land of Canaan a long period of time elapsed, perhaps two or three generations, until unification and the establishment of the new monotheist religion. It is precisely at this moment that traumatic events are most forcefully repressed, removing them from history but not completely destroying them.

Thus, basing himself on the premise of theologian Ernst Sellin, an Old Testament scholar, Freud constructs his hypothesis about the fate of the great leader of the Jewish religion:

> the Jews, who, even by the account in the Bible, were head strong and unruly towards their law-giver and leader, rose against him one day, killed him and threw off the religion of the Aten which had been imposed on them, just as the Egyptians had thrown it off earlier.
>
> (Freud 1939: 60–61)

This is a hypothesis that, for Freud, seemed to be a highly convincing one, as the Egyptian Moses took the same hard line as Akhenaten, imposing his faith in an uncompromising way, and giving orders in perhaps even a stricter way than the pharaoh.

The sacrifices and coercions that Moses's doctrine demanded of his subjects led to a series of revolts against his authority, and it is not hard to imagine some of them being successful and leading to the murder of the great leader as their violent outcome. Consequently, the former Egyptians who murdered Moses repeated via this act what they did not manage to achieve in their thinking. Freud states: "It was a case of 'acting out' instead of remembering, as happens so often with neurotics during the work of analysis" (Freud 1939: 89). In time, the religion that Moses had passed on fell into oblivion, in the same way as Egyptian monotheism did after the death of Akhenaten. The descendants of the Egyptian people tried to wipe out any vestige or trace of the memory of the crime committed against Moses.

As we know, Freud always strived to show that both psychic and social processes are built on the repression of drives or urges. To describe the aetiology of neuroses or psychoses, he identified as series of psychic mechanisms, like repression *[Verdrängung]*, repudiation *[Verwerfung]*, later translated by the French psychoanalyst Jacques Lacan as *foreclosure*, and denial *[Verleugnung]*. Initially used to talk about the constitution of infantile sexuality, denial places the individual in a dual relationship with castration, in which the *knowing* and the *not knowing* about a particular reality both recognize and deny its occurrence. Via denial, individuals manage to reconcile two contradictory beliefs, affirming and denying at the same time two incompatible realities. In this way the truth and lies coexist *simultaneously*.

In *Moses and Monotheism*, Freud elevates denial to the same importance as repression, using it not only to explain the formation of psychic structures, but also to understand the formation of social structures, of the bonds that individuals establish between each other, in a word, of the civilizing process. Civilization is thus constructed on repression as much as on denial and in this way distances itself from each and every disturbing reality. In the case of Jewish monotheism, the murder of Moses after the exodus from Egypt was denied by the Jewish people. Unlike repression, whose content returns as symptoms, dreams and recollections, denial is shifted somewhere else, returning in a distorted way in a new narrative. In the quest to wipe out the traces and memories of this crime, in the attempt to destroy the vestiges of a violent act, trauma resurfaces in a distorted way. Freud writes:

> We might well lend the word "*Entstellung* [distortion]" the double meaning to which it has a claim but of which today it makes no use. It should mean not only "to change the appearance of something" but also "to put something in another place, to displace".
>
> (Freud 1939: 43)

For this reason, Freud reconstructs the narrative of the origins of the Jewish people not based on facts, as history recounts them, but via legends, myths, customs, religions and traditions.

The idea of a single god, highly spiritualized, omnipotent and intolerant of any other god. A religion that demands renouncing drives just as their former leaders demanded of their people. The conviction that the Jews were chosen by God offers the protection and help that they needed. Furthermore, a powerful sense of guilt reproduces the ambivalences inherent in the emotions involved in a relationship with a father that does not permit the expression of hatred and hostility, but only admiration, gratitude and respect. All this constitutes fragments of a truth, as Freud termed it, of a *historical truth* [*historische Wahrheit*]. The return of an attempt to wipe out the murder of Moses. Judaism thus becomes a "religion of the father", re-establishing the lost places of the son and the father via the return of a single God.

Opting to construct a history, just as Freud set out to do in *Moses and Monotheism*, is to claim that understanding the truth is not simply a case of how it corresponds to factual events, seeking to evaluate what is factually "right" and "wrong". Thus right at the start of the second essay, "If Moses Was an Egyptian...", he admits that "even if all the parts of a problem seem to fit together like the pieces of a jig-saw puzzle, one must reflect that what is probable is not necessarily the truth and that the truth is not always probable" (Freud 1939: 17). Freud applies the same approach to the story of Moses as he did for many years to his patients, revealing a hidden truth that lies beyond what is clearly stated.

Consequently, Betty Fuks states: "Freud wants to assert what is unspoken, uncover what is repressed, give a voice to the excluded, in sum prevent one truth exerting its power over another" (2000: 89). *Historical truth* thus becomes a research methodology for exploring psychic and social processes that is not bound by the rigorous, univocal and closed analysis of factual events, since it recognizes in them not only ruptures and discontinuities, but also distortions and transformations. This methodology goes beyond rational explanations, opening up the possibilities of meanings, their multiple significations, and suspending the antithesis between "true" and "false". Historical truth stems from constructions that need to be deciphered, a repressed, hidden reality that must be revealed. Historical truth is the insistence of the repetition of reality on the unconscious. A reality of the past that insists on returning in the present in a distorted way. In other words, historical truth acquires its value as it transmits the return of a past event that cannot have been worked thought due to its traumatic or violent nature. To quote Freud,

> When Moses brought the people the idea of a single god, it was not a novelty but signified the revival of an experience in the primaeval ages of the human family which had long vanished from men's conscious memory. But it had been so important and had produced or paved the way for such deeply penetrating changes in men's life that we cannot avoid believing that it had left behind it in the human mind some permanent traces, which can be compared to a tradition.
>
> (Freud 1939: 129)

Freud thus moves away from historicism that seeks to establish unequivocal truths based on concrete facts. This is, after all, a truth that cannot be proven by events. But what is there to guarantee that Freud or anyone who creates constructions based on pieces or fragments of a previous and forgotten history is right and is not moving even further away from the truth? Freud poses this question in the text *Constructions in Analysis*, providing his own answer as follows: "An equally valuable confirmation is implied (expressed this time positively) When the patient answers with an association which contains something similar or analogous to the content of the construction" (Freud 1937: 263). In the case of the practice of psychoanalysis, the truth of construction is revealed more through the associations that patients make based on what was revealed to them and less through confirmations or denials, the "yes" and "no" answers that they provide. In the case of group phenomena, as applies to Freud's work on the history of the Jewish people, Moses is not present to be able to link the resulting constructions. The answer to the question as to how to guarantee that a historical truth is revealing repressed content that has been forgotten by civilization can be found in *Moses and Monotheism*:

> If our account of primaeval history is accepted as on the whole worthy of belief, two sorts of elements will be recognized in religious doctrines and rituals: on the one hand fixations to the ancient history of the family and survivals of it, and on the other hand revivals of the past and returns, after long intervals, of what has been forgotten.
>
> (Freud 1939: 84)

In this way, we can think of myths, legends, religions, and traditions that recount the histories of peoples and civilizations, as carrying with them fragments of a historical truth. For the civilizing process, they become analogous with the symptoms of individuals, like dreams, customs, and habits, that pass on in a distorted and incomplete way the histories of trauma, violence and barbarity and repeat, without individuals knowing their origins or purposes, memories of a past that cannot be remembered or forgotten.

Tradition, then, retrieves times of harmony, prosperity and progress to mask a past that does not present itself entirely as such. To quote Freud's words, that lead us to think about the work that Norbert Elias created in his biography about the German State:

> Long-past ages have a great and often puzzling attraction for men's imagination. Whenever they are dissatisfied with their present surroundings-and this happens often enough-they turn back to the past and hope that they will now be able to prove the truth of the unextinguishable dream of a golden age. They are probably still under the spell of their childhood, which is presented to them by their not impartial memory as a time of uninterrupted bliss.
>
> (Freud 1939: 71)

Traditions thus become substitute narratives that help remove from memory certain traumatic events, as if they had never happened. In order to repair the present. They retrieve some trace of the past as if they could repair the present time. A fantastical invention structured like fiction. Freud thus continues the above quote as follows:

> If all that is left of the past are the incomplete and blurred memories which we call tradition, this offers an artist a peculiar attraction, for in that case he is free to fill in the gaps in memory according to the desires of his imagination and to picture the period which he wishes to reproduce according to his intentions.
>
> (Freud 1939: 71)

Individuals tend to hide truths whenever they consider them unsatisfactory, inadequate, or incoherent, creating idealized, unreal images to take their place. Norbert Elias, in turn, does not shy away from thinking about how this defence mechanism also operates in social structures. For Para Elias, collective fantasies play an important part as well in the formation of nation-states. In his paper to commemorate the fortieth anniversary of the end of World War II, entitled *Humana Condition*, he refers to the *social myth* as the expression of the egotism of societies, a way of concealing the reality of the barbarities committed by the Third Reich to satisfy a nation's need to assert itself. Elias writes,

> I know there are quite a number of Germans who say: "I don't want to hear any more of all that." But that's the wrong approach. Hitler and his deeds do not disappear from the memory of mankind because they are no longer spoken of. The strong tendency to come to terms with the past through repression leads, I think, to the impossibility of coming to terms with it.
>
> (Elias 1985: 117)

Talking about violent acts and atrocities committed in the past is a way of working through and, consequently, preventing its repetition in the future. In the opinion of Elias, the task of sociology, which we also recognize as one of the purposes of psychoanalysis, is to confront traumas, as he explains below:

> Nothing is more dangerous than the tendency to avoid such a reality by concealing or repressing it. Only when you face it with all courage and determination can you ask the question: What to do in such a situation? And that is indeed the crucial question.
>
> (Elias 1985: 118)

References

Elias, Norbert (1985) "Humana Conditio", in *Collected Works of Norbert Elias – The Loneliness of the Dying and Humana Conditio*, vol. 6, trans. by E. Jephcott. Dublin: University College of Dublin Press, 1991.

——— (1989) *The Germans. Power Struggles and the Development of Habitus in the Nineteenth and Twentieth Centuries*, trans. by E. Dunning and S. Mennell. New York: Columbia University Press, 1996.

Freud, Sigmund (1909) "Family Romances", in *The Standard Edition of the Complete Psychological Works of Sigmund Freud – Jensen's 'Gradiva' and Other Works (1906–1908)*, vol. IX, ed. and trans. by J. Strachey. London: The Hogarth Press, 1981.
——— (1913) "Totem and Taboo", in *The Standard Edition of the Complete Psychological Works of Sigmund Freud – Totem and Taboo and Other Works (1913–1914)*, vol. XIII, ed. and trans. by J. Strachey. London: The Hogarth Press, 1981.
——— (1921) "Group Psychology and the Analysis of the Ego", in *The Standard Edition of the Complete Psychological Works of Sigmund Freud – Beyond the Pleasure Principle, Group Psychology and Other Works (1920–1922)*, vol. XVIII, ed. and trans. by J. Strachey. London: The Hogarth Press, 1981.
——— (1923) "The Ego and the Id", in *The Standard Edition of the Complete Psychological Works of Sigmund Freud – The Ego and the Id and Other Works (1923–1925)*, vol. XIX, ed. and trans. by J. Strachey. London: The Hogarth Press, 1981.
——— (1937) "Construction in Analysis", in *The Standard Edition of the Complete Psychological Works of Sigmund Freud, Volume XXIII (1937–1939): Moses and Monotheism, An Outline of Psychoanalysis and Other Works*, vol. XXIII, ed. and trans. by J. Strachey. London: The Hogarth Press, 1981.
——— (1939) "Moses and Monotheism", in *The Standard Edition of the Complete Psychological Works of Sigmund Freud, Volume XXIII (1937–1939): Moses and Monotheism, an Outline of Psychoanalysis and Other Works*, vol. XXIII, ed. and trans. by J. Strachey. London: The Hogarth Press, 1981.
——— (1986) *The Complete Letters of Sigmund Freud to Wilhelm Fliess: 1887–1904*, ed. and trans. by J. M. Masson. London: Harvard University Press.
——— (1992) *The Diary of Sigmund Freud – 1929–1939: A Record of the Final Decade*, trans. by M. Molnar. New York: Macmillan Publishing Company.
Freud, Sigmund and Ferenczi, Sándor (2000) *The Correspondence of Sigmund Freud and Sándor Ferenczi (1920–1933)*, vol. 3, ed. by E. Falzeder and V. Brabant, trans. by P. Hoffer. London: The Belknap Press of Harvard University Press.
Freud, Sigmund and Zweig, Arnold (1970) *The Letters of Sigmund Freud and Arnold Zweig*, ed. by E. Freud, trans. by E. and W. Robson-Scott. New York: A Harvest Book.
Frosh, Stephen (1987) *The Politics of Psychoanalysis. An Introduction to Freudian and Post-Freudian Theory*. London: MacMillan Press.
Fuks, Betty (2000) *Freud e a judeidade: a vocação do exílio*. Rio de Janeiro: Jorge Zahar.

8 Norbert Elias, beyond Sigmund Freud

The influence of Sigmund Freud's thinking on the work of Norbert Elias is well established and does not need to be demonstrated. But we also know that Elias did not refrain from formulating some critiques of psychoanalysis. Freud, according to Elias, was the heir to modern science and was restricted to Cartesian dualisms that separate the mind from the body, the interior world from the exterior one, nature and culture, subject and object. Consequently, Freud conceived of a given, dated personality structure, in other words, an ahistorical and universal one, without taking into consideration the transformations and changes in societies, or the effects of these on the structure of the psyche. By defining the limits of psychoanalysis, Elias sought to go *beyond Freud*, highlighting that the dynamics of the unconscious and the economy of drives must be described in accordance with the historical and social processes of each society. Elias also illustrated that the psychic structures that are part of Freudian nosology, such as neuroses, psychoses and perversions, are expressions of a social grammar of psychic suffering. He demonstrated that the unconscious, instead of being reduced to each individual's particular conflicts, passes on across the generations collective experiences that manifest themselves as symptom and *social habitus*.

Norbert Elias thus took on the task of historicizing psychoanalysis. What marks our identity does not only relate to affective relationships with family members or those close to us. We are also made up of wider collective experiences, those of the social classes and groups that we belong to, and of our relationship with the country where we were born or live. This is an idea that Freud had already put forward in his 1921 text, *Group Psychology and the Analysis of the Ego*, where he states: "Each individual therefore has a share in numerous group minds – those of his race, of his class, of his creed, of his nationality, etc." (Freud 1921: 129). In other words, we are marked by our society's histories, such that we can consider our identity as the collection of identifications that we construct throughout our live. Freud, however, did not explore the social dimension of psychic suffering in greater depth, limiting his research above all to individual processes within the family sphere. It was Norbert Elias who in fact returned to the imbrication of social structures with psychic ones, dealing with them as different aspects of the same object.

We could consider the text *Freud's concept of society and beyond it* as one of the most important contemporary critiques of Freud's thinking. Written in 1990, it

DOI: 10.4324/9781003378938-8

remained unfinished due to the death of Elias. By then blind, unable to write on his own and obliged to dictate his ideas to his students, this was the final work of a man, that in the words of Bernard Lahire, can be considered "the most Freudian of sociologists" (2010: 35). In it, Elias returns to Freud as a tribute to the thinker that had the greatest influence on him in his life. Discussing, for the first time directly and systematically the ideas and concepts of psychoanalysis, this text can also be understood as Elias's last will and testament, which insists on the importance of considering the interconnections between social and psychic processes, knowing that the unwise inadvertent choice of just one of the elements of this equation can lead to irreparable damage.

8.1 Freudian antagonisms

Norbert Elias fiercely takes issue with the disciplines that establish insurmountable barriers between antithetical terms and that understand them as elements whose existences are separate from each other, as if they were autonomous, independent entities. His intention is to overcome the exclusionary opposition "*either* one *or* the other", proposing an imbrication in which the two elements mutually influence each other, each one causing changes in the other. Thus, in *The Society of Individuals*, he presents his research project as follows: "But what if a better understanding of the relation of individual and society could only be attained by breaking through the either/or, melting the frozen antithesis?" (Elias 1987b: 09).

The antithesis between these terms is not natural and can only be understood in a social context. According to the text *Changes in the We-I Balance* (Elias 1987a), there have been times when individuals' identities verged much more towards collectivity, such that the *we-identity* weighed much heavier than the *self-identity*. Analysis of the civilizing process has shown that the relation between the terms "individual", as a distinctive mark that is not common to everyone, and "society", considered a collection of features shared by a group of people, experiences imbalances that can determine the way we understand and relate these terms. However, the individual and society must be considered as two sides of the same coin, two functions of the same structure.

In *Freud's concept of society*, Elias approaches the sociology of psychoanalysis, underlining that the two disciplines should work with a conceptualization of the individual and of society as entities in constant transformation. "Sociology and psychoanalysis, as I understand them, have in common that they take as a point of departure a dynamic concept – the human being as a process" (Elias 1990: 131), Elias writes. However, Freud was not able to advance any further with this project. He did not grasp the way that changes in society can transform the psychic economy and dynamics, nor how shifts in the personality structure are bound up with social changes. For Norbert Elias Freudian theory and practice therefore remain fundamentally dualistic.

Whatever the discipline, the assumption that there is a stable, complete and independent system ends up being reflected in the way the human condition is thought about. Therefore, the individual sees themselves as "closed personality", self-contained, separated from all others and universally replicable. We encounter this line of thinking in philosophy, where the *homo philosophicus* is not seen as a being whose life has evolved through childhood to the adult stage or even through the historical development of societies. This image of the epistemic individual is accompanied by those of the *homo œconomicus, homo psychoanalyticus, homo historicus* and *homo sociologicus*, defined by the figure that Norbert Elias called the *homo clausus*, whose nucleus, his being, his true self appears to be separated by an invisible wall from everything that is external to them, including all other human beings. The nature of this insurmountable wall has never been the focus of these disciplines. What separates the internal from the external is already a given and established as a self-evident element of the human condition itself.

According to Stephen Mennell (1989), the concept of *homo clausus* relates to the idea of a person, the expression of the universal in the singular, a "subject" of knowledge, a single thinking mind within a closed container, from where it looks outwards and strives to get to know the outside "objects" present in the "external world". Among these objects are other minds, equally closed off within their own containers. One of the greatest difficulties for epistemologists is the question of how a thinking "subject" can get to know something from their cloistered position. However, this model does not allow us to understand the continuity between the personality structure and the social one.

The solution that Elias puts forward, Mennell continues, is to think of the image of the individual as an open being, an *homines aperti*, "tracing the changes in the structure of personality hand in hand with the changes in the structure of human relations in society as part of a global process" (1989: 193), as in the words of his disciple. In this way, Elias concerns himself with investigating the transformation processes of societies over the centuries, the changes in the patterns of civilization, the development of habits and emotions. To do so, his thinking had to turns its back on static positions.

> The image of the human being as a "closed personality" is here replaced by the image of the human being as an "open personality" who possesses a greater or lesser degree of relative (but never absolute and total) autonomy vis-a-vis other people and who is, in face, fundamentally orientated towards and dependent on other people throughout his or her life.
>
> (Elias 1968: 481)

Thus, in *Freud's concept of society*, Elias asks: "What was it that bonded individuals to each other so that they formed social groupings of various kinds?" (1990: 15). Of course, "What binds the individuals together is not cement", he says, jokingly, in *The Society of Individuals* (1987b: 13). But what elements make it possible for individual to coexist with each other, establishing different types of relationships with each other? It is not due to a gregarious instinct, nor the desire for a sovereign or due to a social contract that people get close to each other. In *Sociology and Psychiatry*, Elias writes, referencing Freudian theory: "Some current theories give the impression that only valency is, as it were, beamed from one individual towards another, the sexual valency]" (Elias 1969: 131). In other words, neither can we simply reduce to sexual interests the reason why people meet up in the most diverse spaces forming the most different kinds of relationships. The forces that drive a human being towards another are numerous and varied.

According to Elias, every person, within their network of social relations, has a place, a function, taking on some kind of task for others. The concept of function relates to the relational nature of the actions of individuals determined by the power that they hold over each other. In the book *What is Sociology?* [*Was ist Soziologie?*], he states: "Here, as can be seen, the term 'function' is not used as an expression for a task performed by a section within a harmonious 'whole'". (1970a: 77). It should be understood, above all, as a concept of relationship. To avoid function being unilateral and, therefore, no longer thinking in terms of implications from one point to another – for example, society determining from outside the actions of an individual –, Elias states that function is a multi-vector relationship where we find the mutual wielding of power by one person over another:

> We depend on others; others depend on us. In so far as we are more dependent on others than they are on us, more directed by others than they are by us, they have power over us, whether we have become dependent on them by their use of naked force or by our need to be loved, our need for money, healing, status, a career, or simply for excitement.
>
> (Elias 1970a: 93)

Norbert Elias therefore proposes that we think about a structure that should be understood as a configuration of relationships of interdependence, avoiding approaches that take up only one of these terms, *either* individual *or* society. These disjunctions convey the false conceptualizations of individual freedom and social determinism. It is neither one nor the other. Neither is the individual totally free, nor totally determined by external forces or by drives and desires. Elias explains as follows: "For their actions and ideas cannot be explained and understood within the framework of the game" (1970a: 96). Like in a game of chess, the individual players do not have total freedom of choice in a configuration. First, there are rules that organize the game, and second, the history of the game itself determines how the game unfolds.

For Elias, the division between individual and society results from the rationality of the thinking of the modern Western world. In addition to suspending this antithesis, the concept of configuration also impacts on the ideas of *causality*, on what mobilizes the establishment of social ties, and of *power*, that establishes the forces and the tensions that shape the relationship. Power is not about possession, something that the strongest individual possesses to dominate the weakest. Rather, it is a particular feature of all human relationships.

The concept of power, as he proposes, "it is a structural characteristic of huma relationships – of *all* human relationships" (Elias 1970a: 74). Power results from the encounter of social functions. It is not an attribute that can be possessed by isolated components. Power is structural and relational and therefore cannot be qualified as either good or bad. Neither is it an exclusive characteristic of situations of dominance, such as the relation between master and enslaved. On the contrary, it takes on various forms and can be found at all levels of relationships – familial, political, economic, religious. With this conclusion, Elias dismantles the traditional logic between the dominant and the dominated.

In the section on the problems of human interdependences, in the book *What is Sociology?*, Norbert Elias highlights at least three forms of interdependence between individuals. His critiques are first aimed at the theories that do not consider the biological characteristics of human beings as essential elements for the formation of social links. The primordial condition of the physical *unpreparedness* and psychic helplessness of human beings are presented as a fundamental element for our understanding of how individuals approach others and form networks of interdependent relationships. In *The Society of Individuals*, he states: "Only in relation to other human beings does the wild, helpless creature which comes into the world become the psychologically developed person with the character of an individual and deserving the name of an adult human being" (1987b: 21). The notion of helplessness is no stranger to psychoanalysis. Freud used it to qualify the primordial nature of the development of individuals' urges, what makes them look for love and protection in the people who are responsible for their early care.

Still on the subject of interdependences, Elias underlines political and economic links as elements that make possible the establishment of configurations. Extending Weber's line of thought about the state as a social unit who monopolizes the violence, individuals come together in larger groups with the aim of defending their lives and surviving attacks from other groups. The economic monopoly is closely associated with the monopoly of physical violence. According to Elias, Karl Marx was a thinker who was sensitive to this since he understood that the economy is described as an action of the state to protect the interests of a particular social class. The stability of merchants and their properties, the fulfilment of contracts and rates of commercialization between industries – was something that should be suppressed, leading Marx to think about the economy as an autonomous sphere in relation to the state sphere, in other words, the economy follows its own laws.

Even though Elias recognizes that Freud managed to identify a lacuna in traditional sociological theory by stating that social psychology and the psychology of individuals cannot be separated and that, for psychoanalysis, the relationship with others has a central role in the development and constitution of every individual, "The Freudian model of an individual is eminently sociological, his model of society is eminently individualistic" (Elias 1990: 17). According to this statement from Elias, for psychoanalysis, the individual is constituted in the form of a complex of identifications with others, "a society in miniature" (Elias 1990: 17), and society presents itself as an atomistic structure, like the masses, following the same logic of individual psychic processes. Reifying the individual, Freud, Elias argues, conceived of society as a complete structure and of psychic entities as static objects.

Freud's difficulty in understanding social processes stemmed, according to Elias, from his investment in therapeutic practice, which led him to be interested only in the psychic suffering of individuals. Even if Freud had been open to a sociological explanation of the experiences of individuals, he would not have been able to grasp the social identity of individuals, their *we-identity*. Says Elias: "His [Freud] whole concept formation was centred on the first person singular. Concepts such as ego, superego and ego ideal are characteristic of Freud's productivity, but also of his limitations" (Elias 1990: 18). Freud, therefore, was a thinker of his time and expressed, in the formulation of his theory and his concepts, the conflicts of his time. For Elias, psychoanalytical theory, centred exclusively on the "ego", leads to an unbalanced vision between the levels of the "ego" and of the "we". Neither was Freud careful in differentiating the repressive characteristics of societies through the ages. In his view, it is as if repression had always existed.

The distinction between the individual and society resurfaces in Freud, according to Elias, in diverse antagonisms. Elias writes,

> In one of the most telling expressions of his view, he [Freud] linked the antagonism between individual and society to that between Eros and Thanatos, between the fulfilling love-drive with all its ramifications and what he had come to regard as its eternal opponent, the human drive towards destruction and death.
>
> (1990: 20)

At several points in his work Freud pointed out differences between the psychic reality, ruled by the pleasure principles and drives, and the external reality, organized around the principle of social coercions and reality, and, in texts like *The Loss of Reality in Neurosis and Psychosis* (Freud 1924), he explained the formation of psychic structures (neurosis and psychosis) as a conflict with reality. As a consequence, in *Sociology and Psychiatry*, Elias stated that "many of Freud's theoretical concepts suggest the existence of a wall between the 'internal' fantasies which he explored and the 'external' reality which he did not explore" (1969: 137). It is as if neuroses allow individuals to see in the external world only what they end up transferring of themselves, in the form of fantasy. In the case of psychoses, on the other hand, reality is recreated in the form of delusions and hallucinations.

According to Elias, Freud also, in his opinion, upheld the distinction between nature and culture, animality and humanity. In *Freud's concept of society*, Elias underlined the problematic ambivalence of these terms: "Freud believed that life in society runs counter to human nature" (1990: 27) and, furthermore, stated that Freud considered society "the eternal antagonist of the individual human being" (1990: 28). Basing himself on the definition of culture put forward in *Civilization and Its Discontents*, as the sum total of achievements and regulations which distinguish our lives in society from those of our animal ancestors, Elias is able to conclude that: "He saw humans only as something more than animals, not also as beings evolved from animals into something else" (1990: 47). For Elias, defence mechanisms and psychic structures of self-control, such as the ego, the superego and the ego ideal, according to psychanalysis, result from the relationship of individuals in society, whereas the libido and drives are expressions of animal instincts. One is the antagonist of the other. Whereas drives, in his view, are manifestations of nature, higher psychic mechanisms originate from social relations, and are a manifestation that is *anti-nature*.

In this sense, Freud inherited a metaphysical stance, in Elias's view, establishing distinctions between what stems from animal nature and what stems from human nature. However, Elias writes: "They [human beings] are by their very nature constituted for life in groups. There is no zero-point, no beginning where individuals who live alone for one reason or another decide to form groups or societies with each other" (1990: 48). It is here that the sociologist differs from Freud. It is also here that his project to historicize psychoanalysis and reinterpret Freudian concepts, seeing psychic structures as political, historical and social expressions, emerges.

8.2 The myth of origins and the civilizing process

The use of certain words leads to descriptions that restrict themselves to relationships of opposition: subject versus object, internal world versus external world, ego versus the other, nature versus culture. Language obliges us to speak and think as if these elements were isolated, static entities, without considering them in relation to each other. More than elaborations of great philosophical works, these antitheses have been embedded in our way of thinking through the way in which we behave and speak in our daily lives. The geocentric vision, that is still rooted in daily expressions like "sunrise" or "sunset", a vestige of an era when human beings could not yet establish a distance from themselves, is an example of a logic of thought that remains in our language. When we refer to someone and describe them as an individual isolated from their environment, independent of others and distanced from their history, we are also making explicit the way in which we understand human beings. With these statements we exclude the development processes that person has gone through, their relationships with those closest to them, and the places they occupy within the various social groups they are part of. We therefore assume that we can dominate ourselves, control our origins and project our future.

The specificity of sociological theories – and this could be extended to any realm of thinking that investigates human relationships – results not from the object we are examining but from the concepts we are drawing on. To move away from the non-relational, fragmented conceptualization of elements in a particular configuration – whatever the degree of complexity, like in a card game or 16th-century French court society –, it is necessary to renounce not just linguistic resources used in daily life, but also the specialized language used in scientific and academic thinking. This is also the case with terms like state, school, family, child, and person. Taking them as independent terms distances them from any relationships that they establish and positions them as social antitheses. It is as if a child's behaviour only has to do with the child themselves and is not an effect of the place they occupy within a complex network of relationships, or as if their parents did not need to abide by the resolutions of society and the state.

Norbert Elias's intellectual project seeks to distance itself from certain traditional hegemonic ways of thinking that are characterized as: *metaphysical*, that substantiate beings as if they existed autonomously and independently; *dualistic*, that think about relationships as if they were dichotomies expressed in terms of cause and effect, subject and object, interior and exterior; *teleological*, that see processes as if they were the visible evolution of the fulfilment of a particular objective; *normative*, that aim towards a scientificity in which the researcher considers themselves excluded from their research object; *deterministic*, that need to correlate the formation of effects to the mechanistic necessity of a cause; *fragmentary*, that think about the world in a discontinuous way as being constituted by particular elements closed off from others.

In an interview with Johan Goudsblom, Norbert Elias responds as follows to the question about the status of Freudian theory: "But psycho-analysis, while it was an enormous breakthrough, has a theoretical framework which is also an example of *Zustandsreduktion*" (Elias 1970b: 137). What he means here is the psychoanalysis remains a theory that produces as *processual reduction*, in other words, a reduction of a process to a state or also the separation between the individual and their objects of relation. When Goudsblom replies that, even so, Elias drew on psychoanalysis in its theoretical and dynamic senses, Elias continues this critique: "Yes, but psychoanalysts often proceed as if e.g. super-ego structures were unchanging. Further developments of psycho-analytic theory will be necessary for the practical problems which I have raised", then restating: "My own friends who are psycho-analysts realize that psycho-analysts will have to collaborate far more with sociologists in the future than is the case today. There is no fruitful way to further development of psycho-analytic theory except by interdisciplinary collaboration" (Elias 1970b: 137).

Following this line of thought, Sabine Delzescaux identifies three characteristics of Elias's sociology. First, as *multi-dimensional sociology*, it situates its main object, human beings, within a set of complex integrations. As well as being made up of flesh and blood, they are also historical beings, who are localized in a particular time and space, and thinking beings, that act and are acted upon in accordance with different kinds of social organization. The second characteristic of Norbert Elias's sociology, according to Delzescaux, refers to *multi-disciplinarity*. The study of the transformations of individuals and societies presupposes a knowledge that is not limited to that of sociology: "sociological knowledge cannot be considered properly sociological insofar as it feeds on the contributions of disciplines as diverse as philosophy, history, psychoanalysis, or even biology" (2001: 32). Finally, Elias's sociology is marked by *processuality*. The concept of process is perhaps one of the most important in Elias's work – to that extent that the latter is considered a processual sociology –inscribing in his research the transformations and changes of social structures and their psychic counterparts without needing to resort to a starting point or an end point.

The study of the past is an essential issue both for Sigmund Freud and Norbert Elias. But, unlike Elias, whose research focuses on long-term processed without beginnings, for psychoanalysis the question of the origin of humanity plays a central role. Elias writes: "Like Hobbes and the social contract philosophers, Freud asked about the beginning of Society" (1990: 22). Freud's response also draws on the contractualist philosophy of Thomas Hobbes, according to which violence – first by the father, then by murderous sons and finally by the entire group against every individual – is considered the cause of the formation of societies. But for the sociologist, the idea of a point of origin of collective life ultimately separates nature from culture, the individuals from society, biological conditions from learning experiences.

In *Totem and Taboo*, Freud (1913) presents the beginning of society via the fictional narrative of the primal horde. According to this narrative, in a mythical time there was a group led by an older man who was supposedly stronger and enjoyed the privileges of relations with women. On the one hand, the members of the horde felt protected and loved by the leader. Subjected to the tyranny of this strongest figure, they were forbidden from satisfying their urges and emotions. On the other hand, the father of the horde was located beyond social relationships. He was subject to no kind of coercion or regulation. However, on a particular day, the brothers who were expelled from the horde joined forces, killed their father and devoured his body. Once united, they achieved what each of them, individually, would not have done. Based on this primary act, they put an end to the tyranny of the sovereign, transferred his power to the community and began to organize themselves into a society ruled by codes and norms that gave rise to law and justice.

For Freud, the passage of the primal horde, in which at least one is free of social coercions, to fraternal organization, in which everyone is equal, is explained by the collective murder of the father. This mythical act, the foundation of civilization, is what distances the individual from their natural impulses. It establishes socially shared habits, rules and codes and, therefore, is considered by Freud as the origin of social institutions. To preserve civilization and avoid the return to the state of barbarity of the primal horde, no isolated individual could take the place of the absolute, sovereign leader. By identifying with the dead father, the members of the horde introject this authority figure in the form of psychic structures of self-control, like the superego and the ego ideal.

These explanations thus return to a comparison of the two authors. Freud proposed the beginning of civilization as the murder of an all-powerful individual, chief of the horde, free of any kind of social coercion whatsoever. Elias states from the outset that this would be impossible, since any individual, to be able to survive, needs the protection and safety of a group. Those who seek some kind of isolation end up in extremely vulnerable positions and are unable to survive for long. Further, in the sociologist's thinking, "Yet there is no point in time known or even imaginable at which human beings without society submitted themselves, freely or by force, to the rule of society" (Elias 1990: 22).

Questions about the beginning of society gave rise to many scientific myths and legends, of which the Freudian hypothesis of the parricide of the primal horde is just one example. A mythological inclination that can be understood as a theoretical reductionism based on limited information and, above all, on an inappropriate conceptual framework. Elias does not fail to observe that Freud's theory of society is a product of a time when we were not yet in a position to see society structured as a whole. From this perspective, the hypothesis of the primal horde bears the mark of *autonomy* and of *exclusion*, as if the existence of individuals outside society and of societies outside individuals were possible. The Freudian concept of society, Elias writes, is nothing more than an antagonism of human nature.

In this way the sociologist turns into a veritable "destroyer of myths" (Elias 1970a), since "Freud might not have felt the need for inventing his myth of the primeval band of brothers, a more colourful rehash of the social contract theory, if he had accepted the evolutionary model of the origins of society" (1990: 26). There is no good reason, according to Elias, for us to reject the statement that human societies evolved from animal societies, in a continuous process through which our ancestors were transformed until they arrived at their current state.

Elias argues that it is necessary to move away from the need for a "point of departure", often the point of departure of the individual themselves, to be able to recognize the influence of processual and longitudinal elements. In Elias's vision, the capacity for individual self-control resulted from a long process of social learning that occurred over many centuries. A single traumatic event, that allegedly occurred millennia ago and that is considered as the absolute beginning of society and civilization, overlooks all the learning experiences, social transformations and changes in the psychic economy of individuals. Here is the difference: for Elias, there is no beginning, there is no origin; for Freud, everything began with an act.

In Elias's view, Freud was also unable to explain the transmission process of collective experiences, like this mythical event, leaning more towards phylogenetic explanations, of an innate nature, than to processual ones, relating to learning. Norbert Elias underlines the role of personal pronouns as determinants of the place of the speech of individuals throughout civilizing processes: "It leads people to believe that their actual 'selves' somehow exist 'inside' them; and that an invisible barrier separates their 'inside' from everything 'outside' – the so-called 'outside world'" (Elias 1970a: 119). The use of personal pronouns normally confers on their referents the quality of nouns. The pronoun "I", for example, when treated as an object of study, is transformed into a substance, into an independent thing, while the pronouns "you" and "he/they" are like other entities to the former. But it is impossible to refer to the singular person excluding them from the plurality of their relations and from the place they occupy in these configurations. According to the logic of the games model, Elias's critique again refers to the individualizing use of these pronouns: "The function of the pronoun 'I' in human communication can only be understood in the context of all the other positions to which the other terms in the series refer" (Elias 1970a: 123). Thus Elias questions the barrier that shuts off human beings in isolated and independent entities (*homo clausus*), to present them instead as diverse interdependent "Is", with valences open to the different ways of building social ties.

When treated as functions, personal pronouns prove to be intrinsically relational, such that we cannot think of the "I", without the "you", "he/they" and "we". These pronouns indicate the collection of coordinates used to represent societies or any kind of human plurality. The "I", from where you speak to the "you", is included in the "we" as its collective, leaving the "he/they" with the role located outside the group: "Taken together, the personal pronouns are in fact an elementary expression of the fact that every person is fundamentally related to other people, and that every human individual is fundamentally a social being (1970a: 124). It is impossible to talk about "we" without conceiving of the "I" from where the individual addressed the "he/they".

These are basic positions that situate the relationships between diverse configurations, whether of the individual who speaks "for themselves" or "for the group" they belong to. This suggests that the sole individual refers to a person in relationships of interdependence and society, in turn, refers to the collection of people in relationships of interdependence. Consequently, with the use of personal pronouns as a model for thinking about configurations, we can grasp how it is possible to think about a *distinction* between research about people in the singular and research about people in the plural, but it is impossible to separate them, just as singular persons cannot be separated from plural persons. Internal world and external world, individual and society, I and other, subject and object, civilization and nature, public and private, all these antithetical terms, when considered in themselves, do not mean anything and nor do they have specific objects. It is necessary to formulate a terminology that indicates more clearly the specificity of the relation between dichotomous terms. In fact, new theoretical and conceptual models will be needed to break down the barriers between the sciences.

In Freudian theory, as Elias illustrates, there is a lack of understanding that the concept of the ego and superego do not only refer to individual self-control mechanisms, but also to a way of constructing collective identities, via which the members of a group differentiate themselves from members of another group, or also within the group itself, considering their stage of development. In other words: "'Ego' and 'superego', in other words, are not only aspects of a person's individual habitus, but also of a person's social habitus" (Elias 1990: 45). Therefore, if Freud showed that individuals reveal their conflicts via symptoms and dreams, Norbert Elias went further and demonstrated that habits and customs, unconsciously reproduced by individuals, without them realizing this, are also ways of passing on conflicts. For Elias, habits are the soil from where the personal characteristics of an individual sprout "a more or less individual style, what might be called an unmistakable individual handwriting that grows out of the social script" (1987a: 182). But habits are also social formations that can be considered homologous to the formations of the unconscious. We know about our habits, our dreams and our symptoms, but we do not know why we repeat them nor what they mean. Thus we can say that symptoms, dreams and *social habitus* reproduce social conflicts in the singularity of every individual.

In *Freud's concept of society*, Elias sets out to present further re-readings of psychoanalytical concepts in the light of processual sociology. The libido and urges, defence mechanisms like repression, as well as psychic structures like the id, the ego, the superego and the *ego ideal*, are positioned within social transformations. Even the way that Freud describes the concept of "unconscious", undoubtedly one of the main pillars of psycho-analytical theory, is criticized to the extent that Elias bluntly states: "It is possible to present Freud's finding without using the term 'the unconscious'" (Elias 1990: 42). For Elias, the way Freud presents his concepts does not free him from certain dichotomies.

There is thus a need to bring about a new Copernican revolution to reconfigure the relationship between subject and object. Antitheses like "inside *or* outside", "your own *or* another's", "me *or* the other", "nature *or* culture" and "individual *or* society" are suspended when we begin situating ourselves within a network of relationships belonging to a socially constructed historical context. Elias sets out to establish a new science, as he describes in *The Society of Individuals*:

> The structures of the human psyche, the structures of human society and the structures of human history are indissolubly complementary, and can only be studied in conjunction with each other. They do not exist and move in reality with the degree of isolation assumed by current research. They form, with other structures, the subject matter of the single human science.
>
> (Elias 1987a: 36)

Elias's critiques focus on the absolutist pretension of certain sciences, which seek to occupy a higher position in relation to other disciplines in an epistemological pedantry that obliges the universality of knowledge, on the one hand, to reject historical processes and dismiss transformations of society, and on the other, to assert the position of the individual as one of total isolation. In their desire for power, the sciences construct definitive, arrogant discourses, obtain the right to privileges and disseminate the narcissistic promise of establishing truths. For Elias, however, neither psychoanalysis nor sociology – nor any other discipline – should insist on their dichotomies, since this runs the risk of reproducing a logic of exclusion that establishes hierarchies of values and imposes the need to uphold one of the sides of the equation without considering the harmful ethical consequences of this decision.

References

Delzescaux, Sabine (2001) *Norbert Elias: une sociologie des processus*. Paris: L'Harmatann.

Elias, Norbert (1968) "Postscript", in *The Civilizing Process*, ed. by E. Dunning, J. Goudsblom and S. Mennell, trans. by E. Jephcott. Oxford: Blackwell Publishing, 2013.

——— (1969) "Sociology and Psychiatry", in *Psychiatry in a Changing Society*, ed. by S. Foulkes and G. S. Prince. London: Routledge, 2002.

——— (1970a) *What is Sociology?*, trans. by S. Mennell and G. Morrissey. London: Hutchinson & Co, 1978.

——— (1970b) "Interview Met Norbert Elias Door Johan Goudsblom", in *Sociologische Gids*, vol. 17, n.2, p. 137. https://ugp.rug.nl/sogi/article/view/21409/18880.

——— (1987a) "Changes in the We-I Balance", in *The Society of Individuals*, ed. by M. Schröter, trans. by E. Jephcott. New York/London: The Continuum International Publishing Group, 2001.

——— (1987b) "The Society of Individuals", in *The Society of Individuals*, ed. by M. Schröter, trans. by E. Jephcott. New York/London: The Continuum International Publishing Group, 2001.

——— (1990) "Freud's Concept of Society and Beyond it", in *Collected Works of Norbert Elias. Supplements and Index of the Collected Works*, vol. 18, ed. by E. Dunning, J. Heilbron, R. van Krieken and S. Mennell. Dublin: University College of Dublin Press, 2010.

Freud, Sigmund (1913) "Totem and Taboo", in *The Standard Edition of the Complete Psychological Works of Sigmund Freud – Totem and Taboo and Other Works (1913–1914)*, vol. XIII, ed. and trans. by J. Strachey. London: The Hogarth Press, 1981.

——— (1921) "Group Psychology and the Analysis of the Ego", in *The Standard Edition of the Complete Psychological Work of Sigmund Freud – Beyond the Pleasure Principle, Group Psychology and Other Works (1920–1922)*, vol. XVIII, ed. and trans. by J. Strachey. London: Hogarth Press, 1981.

——— (1924) "The Loss of Reality in Neurosis and Psychosis", in *The Standard Edition of the Complete Psychological Work of Sigmund Freud – The Ego and the Id and Other Works (1923–1925)*, vol. XIX, ed. and trans. by J. Strachey. London: Hogarth Press, 1981.

Lahire, Bernard (2010) "Freud, Elias and Human Science", in *Norbert Elias and Social Theory*, ed. by F. Dépelteau and T. S. Landini. New York, Palgrave-Macmillan, 2013.

Mennell, Stephen (1989) *Norbert Elias – An Introduction*. Dublin: University College Dublin Press, 1992.

Index

Taylor & Francis Group
an **informa** business

Taylor & Francis eBooks

www.taylorfrancis.com

A single destination for eBooks from Taylor & Francis with increased functionality and an improved user experience to meet the needs of our customers.

90,000+ eBooks of award-winning academic content in Humanities, Social Science, Science, Technology, Engineering, and Medical written by a global network of editors and authors.

TAYLOR & FRANCIS EBOOKS OFFERS:

A streamlined experience for our library customers

A single point of discovery for all of our eBook content

Improved search and discovery of content at both book and chapter level

REQUEST A FREE TRIAL

support@taylorfrancis.com

Routledge
Taylor & Francis Group

CRC Press
Taylor & Francis Group